普通高等教育"十一五"国家级规划教材

全国高等医药院校药学类专业第二轮实验双语教材

天然药物化学实验与指导

（第3版）

主　　编　冯　锋　罗建光
副主编　殷志琦
编　　者　（以姓氏笔画为序）
　　　　　才　谦（辽宁中医药大学）
　　　　　冯　锋（中国药科大学）
　　　　　曲　玮（中国药科大学）
　　　　　杨官娥（山西医科大学）
　　　　　陈佩东（南京中医药大学）
　　　　　罗建光（中国药科大学）
　　　　　柳润辉（海军军医大学）
　　　　　殷志琦（中国药科大学）
　　　　　黄雪峰（中国药科大学）

中国健康传媒集团
中国医药科技出版社

内容提要

　　本教材是"全国高等医药院校药学类专业第二轮实验双语教材"之一。本教材由天然药物化学常用实验方法、天然药物化学实验实例、附录、参考文献组成。其中，天然药物化学实验中常用方法和天然药物化学实验实例这两个核心部分用中英双语编写，以满足天然药物化学实验的双语教学要求，有助于提高学生的专业英语水平。本教材为书网融合教材，即纸质教材有机融合电子教材、教学配套资源（PPT、微课等）、题库系统、数字化教学服务（在线教学、在线作业、在线考试），使教学资源更加多样化、立体化。

　　本教材主要适用于高等医药院校药学类和中药学类本科学生学习使用，也可作为成人教育和自学的参考教材。

图书在版编目（CIP）数据

天然药物化学实验与指导/冯锋，罗建光主编 . — 3 版 . —北京：中国医药科技出版社，2019. 12

全国高等医药院校药学类专业第二轮实验双语教材

ISBN 978 - 7 - 5214 - 1388 - 5

Ⅰ.①天…　Ⅱ.①冯…②罗…　Ⅲ.①生药学 - 药物化学 - 化学实验 - 双语教学 - 医学院校 - 教学参考资料　Ⅳ.①R284 - 33

中国版本图书馆 CIP 数据核字（2020）第 000766 号

美术编辑　陈君杞
版式设计　友全图文

出版　**中国健康传媒集团** | 中国医药科技出版社

地址　北京市海淀区文慧园北路甲 22 号

邮编　100082

电话　发行：010 - 62227427　邮购：010 - 62236938

网址　www. cmstp. com

规格　889 × 1194 mm $\frac{1}{16}$

印张　$9\frac{1}{2}$

字数　212 千字

初版　2003 年 8 月第 1 版

版次　2019 年 12 月第 3 版

印次　2022 年 8 月第 2 次印刷

印刷　三河市万龙印装有限公司

经销　全国各地新华书店

书号　ISBN 978 - 7 - 5214 - 1388 - 5

定价　**29.00 元**

获取新书信息、投稿、为图书纠错，请扫码联系我们。

教学是学校人才培养的中心环节，实验教学是这一环节的重要组成部分。"全国高等医药院校药学类专业实验双语教材"是中国药科大学坚持药学实践教学改革，突出提高学生动手能力、创新思维，通过承担教育部"世行贷款21世纪初高等教育教学改革项目"等多项教改课题，逐步建设完善的一套与药学各专业学科理论课程紧密结合的高水平双语实验教材。

本轮修订，适逢"全国高等医药院校药学类专业第五轮规划教材"及《中国药典》（2020年版）、新版《国家执业药师资格考试大纲》出版，整套教材的修订强调了与新版理论教材知识的结合，与《中国药典》（2020年版）等新颁布的法典法规结合。为更好地服务于新时期高等院校药学教育与人才培养的需要，在上一版的基础上，进一步体现了各门实验课程自身独立性、系统性和科学性，又充分考虑到各门实验课程之间的联系与衔接，主要突出了以下特点。

1. 适应医药行业对人才的要求，体现行业特色，契合新时期药学人才需求的变化，使修订后的教材符合《中国药典》（2020年版）等国家标准及新版《国家执业药师资格考试大纲》等行业最新要求。

2. 更新完善内容，打造教材精品。在上版教材基础上进一步优化、精炼和充实内容。紧密结合"全国高等医药院校药学类专业第五轮规划教材"，强调与实际需求相结合，进一步提高教材质量。

3. 为适应信息化教学的需要，本轮教材全部打造成为书网融合教材，即纸质教材与数字教材、配套教学资源、题库系统、数字化教学服务有机融合，为读者提供全免费增值服务。

4. 坚持双语体系，强调素质培养教材以实践教学为突破口，采用双语体系编写有利于加快药学教育国际接轨，提高学生的科技英语水平，进一步提升学生整体素质。

"全国高等医药院校药学类专业第二轮实验双语教材"历经15年4次建设，在各个时期广大编者的努力下，在广大使用教材师生的支持下日臻完善。本轮教材的出版，必将对推动新时期我国高等药学教育的发展产生积极而深远的影响。希望广大师生在教学实践中对本套教材提出宝贵意见，以便今后进一步修订完善，共同打造精品教材。

吴晓明

全国高等医药院校药学类专业第五轮规划教材常务编委会主任委员

2019年10月

天然药物化学是运用现代科学理论与技术对天然药物的药效物质基础进行化学研究的一门课程。我国天然药物资源十分丰富，达 12800 种以上。天然药物化学是以寻找和发现天然物质中药效活性成分和重要的前导化合物为目的的化学研究，在以天然产物为来源的新药研发中，占有重要的地位。

《天然药物化学实验指导》是天然药物化学的实验课程教材，由天然药物化学常用实验方法、天然药物化学实验实例、附录和参考文献几部分组成。其中，天然药物化学常用实验方法和天然药物化学实验实例这两个核心部分用中英双语编写，以满足天然药物化学实验的双语教学需求，有助于提高学生的专业英语水平。本教材为书网融合教材，即纸质教材有机融合电子教材、教学配套资源（PPT、微课等）、题库系统、数字化教学服务（在线教学、在线作业、在线考试），使教学资源更加多样化、立体化。《天然药物化学实验指导》主要适用于高等医药院校药学类和中药学类本科学生学习使用，也可用作成人教育和自学的参考教材。

本教材由冯锋、罗建光担任主编，并由冯锋负责统稿、审定工作。与前两版相比，本教材修订了实验设计中的问题，添加了柱色谱实验实例，进一步规范、润色了语言。本教材具体编写分工如下："第一部分天然药物化学常用实验方法""第二部分天然药物化学实验实例"中实验一、二由冯锋编写，实验三、十五由殷志琦编写，实验四、九、十二由才谦编写，实验五、十三由曲玮编写，实验六、十七由陈佩东编写，实验七、十四由黄雪峰编写，实验八、十一由杨官娥编写，实验十、十六由柳润辉编写；附录由罗建光编写。

由中国药科大学天然药物化学教研室编写的《天然药物化学实验》讲义应用多年，是全教研室许多教师教学的心血结晶，对本教材的编写具有极为宝贵的参考价值。本教材的编写，得到了所有编者和同行专家的大力支持与帮助，在此一并表示衷心地感谢。

在编写的过程中，我们做了很大努力，但由于编者学术水平和编写能力所限，疏漏与不足之处在所难免，敬请广大师生和读者予以指正。

编　者

2019 年 08 月

第一部分 天然药物化学常用实验方法

一、提取

1. 提取 提取分离是尽量使目标成分和非目标成分分开、去粗取精的过程。植物体内的成分是由多种复杂的化学成分所组成。其中，生物碱、萜类、甾体、黄酮、蒽醌、香豆素、有机酸、氨基酸、单糖、低聚糖、多糖、蛋白质、酶及鞣质等，一般被认为具有药用价值；而纤维素、叶绿素、蜡、油脂、树脂和树胶等，被认为具有经济价值，因此在研究植物生理活性成分时作为杂质除去。这里介绍一些提取分离所需成分、去除杂质的常用方法。

（1）水提取　水提取可分为水煎、水浸和水渗漉三种，也可用酸水或碱水提取。碱性、酸性或苷类化合物，如小檗碱、甘草酸、芦丁等，较易溶于水，可选用水为提取溶剂。但是用水提取时，提取液中杂质较多（如无机盐、蛋白质、糖和淀粉等），不利于进一步分离。因此，有些化合物虽能溶于水，但为了使杂质尽量少带出来，也常常用有机溶剂提取。

（2）有机溶剂提取　有机溶剂提取常采用回流提取法、索氏提取法、浸渍法和渗漉法。可采用几种极性不同的溶剂，由低极性到高极性分步提取，根据各成分在不同极性溶剂中的溶解度差异而进行分离。也可采用单一溶剂提取。而乙醇溶解性能好，对植物细胞的穿透能力强，单一提取的常用溶剂为不同浓度的乙醇－水溶液，浓度则根据被提取物质的性质而定。

（3）水蒸气蒸馏　挥发油和某些挥发性成分能用水蒸气蒸馏得到。如麻黄碱可用水蒸气蒸馏法从麻黄中直接蒸馏出来。

几种常见提取方法的装置见图1-1和图1-2。

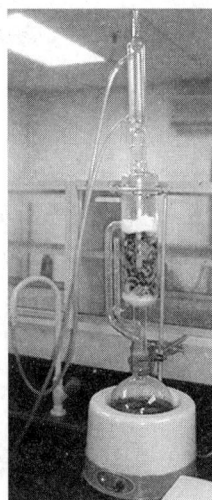

图1-1　索氏提取装置

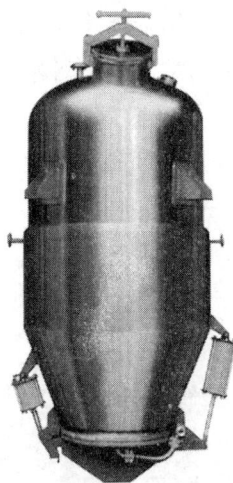

图1-2　渗漉桶

2. 过滤 过滤是从液体中分离固体的简单方法，常用于去除溶液中的不溶物和提取后去除药渣。通常，过滤的操作是通过滤纸和漏斗来实现的，有时也会采用柱过滤。常见的装置见图 1-3。

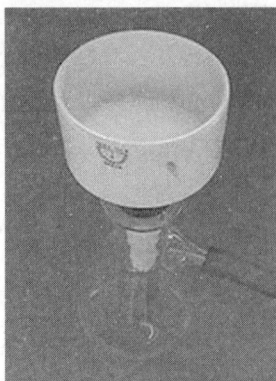

图 1-3 布氏抽滤装置

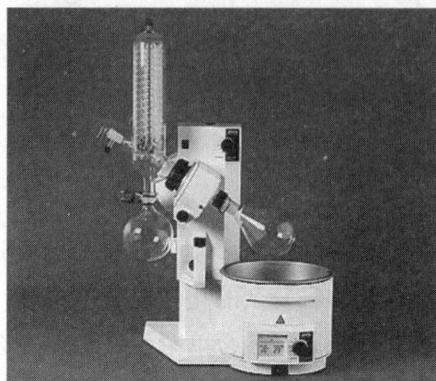

图 1-4 旋转蒸发仪

3. 浓缩 提取液的浓缩通常用旋转蒸发仪和冷冻干燥法。对于绝大多数化学实验室来说，旋转蒸发仪并不陌生，其浓缩过程是将样品溶液在减压条件下降低沸点，而样品的旋转可以使得溶剂蒸发时具有最大的受热面积，溶液的蒸气被冷凝收集于另外的容器中，最后得到的浸膏是圆底烧瓶内壁上的一层薄膜状物。而含有表面活性物质的溶液，在旋转蒸发时容易形成泡沫而冲出容器，有时可以加入少量具有表面活性的有机溶剂（如正丁醇）以减少泡沫的形成。冷冻干燥在高真空度下进行，涉及冷冻后固体水的升华。样品溶液首先用液态二氧化碳或氟利昂冷冻，然后置真空中升华去水。当冷冻干燥中的样品不再失重时，即已干燥。常见装置见图 1-4。

二、分离、纯化方法

1. 萃取/索氏提取/柱过滤等 通常所指的萃取，即液-液分配萃取，是利用混合物中的各成分在两种互不相溶的溶液中分配系数的不同而达到分离的目的。当提取溶剂选用的是水或乙醇-水溶液时，提取后浓缩成浓水液，选择合适的有机溶剂与其萃取。若目标成分是脂溶性，可用亲脂性有机溶剂如石油醚、三氯甲烷或乙醚；若目标成分是亲水性物质，用中等极性溶剂如乙酸乙酯等或亲水性溶剂如正丁醇等。

2. 脱盐、去叶绿素

（1）脱盐 脱盐是分离水溶性成分的一个重要步骤，使其易于分离。脱盐通常是简单的用水和与水不混溶的有机溶剂混合溶解无机盐，借以除去无机盐的步骤。如果有效成分是脂溶性的，可以用反相柱（如 C18 柱）或其他各种有机聚合物（如 XAD-2，XAD-4 和 XAD-7）。用含水溶剂洗脱，盐最先被纯水洗脱，随后其他有效成分被不同浓度的有机溶液洗脱。这种脱盐方法不能用于强极性或离子化合物如极性氨基酸或糖。另一种常用的脱盐方法是排阻柱如葡聚糖凝胶 LH-10 和聚丙烯酰胺凝胶 P-2，但无机离子与化合物及其与柱子间的难以预知的相互作用常改变洗脱的顺序。

在大多数情况下，提取和分馏水溶性化合物必须用缓冲溶液。也就是说，水溶性成分分离的关键是找到合适的 pH 和离子浓度使化合物在给定基质上可分离。然而，缓冲盐和化合物分离很困难，这是因为缓冲盐多为仅有弱离子键作用、减压或冷冻干燥时有挥发性的弱酸和弱碱混合物。但实际上这些缓冲盐并不是很容易处理。

（2）去叶绿素　叶绿素是植物中普遍存在的绿色色素，叶中含量最高，能溶于一般有机溶剂，较难溶于水。水溶液中的叶绿素可用石油醚或三氯甲烷萃取除去。乙醇或乙醇水溶液的提取浓缩液可加水或挥去乙醇至浓度为 15% ~ 20%，冷藏，使叶绿素沉淀出来。另外，叶绿素溶于碱水，不溶于酸水故也可通过酸碱处理除去，使用此法时要求目标成分稳定、且溶于酸水或不溶于碱水。

3. 离心薄层色谱法　经典的制备薄层色谱法有几个缺点，主要缺点是目标化合物在板上刮下时带下的杂质和随后洗脱中带下的吸附剂会对测定产生影响。其他缺点包括分离时间长、存在杂质以及使用溶剂提取目标化合物时吸附剂带有的杂质。

为了克服这些问题，采用了离心色谱法。原则上来讲，离心色谱法的技术是通过经典的 TLC 采用一个离心力的作用加速流动相的流动——一个强化流动的方法。

离心色谱仪（图 1 - 5）与以往色谱仪最大的区别在于它的转轴是倾斜的而非水平的。仪器的核心是直径 24 cm 载有合适吸附剂的用于制备的玻璃圆盘，吸附剂中需要加入黏合剂防止板开裂。多数厚度为 2 mm 的硅胶板可以按下述方法制备：将薄层色谱硅胶 GF_{254}（60g）放入 250 ml 锥形瓶中，加入 180 ml 0.8% 的 CMC - Na，剧烈振摇后，将适量调好的吸附剂倒在玻璃板上，铺板。室温干燥后置烘箱（60 ~ 70℃）活化 30 min，冷却后，用固定在金属盘上的刮刀使吸附剂表面平滑，玻璃板中央有一小部分面积空出以便于引入流动相。另外，还使用加硝酸银的硅胶或氧化铝做吸附剂。

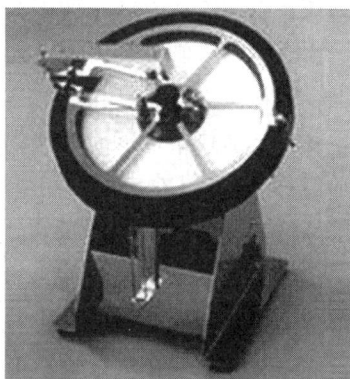

图 1 -5　离心薄层色谱仪

制备好的板（固定相厚度 1、2 或 4 mm）固定在电机的转轴上，流动相从圆盘中心没有固定相处，经泵以 1 ~ 10ml/min 流速导入，在重力作用下经过薄层板，首先洗去吸附剂上的杂质。接着，上样或烘干后上样，再用流动相洗脱。

旋转部分被放在以石英玻璃覆盖的腔内，这样对那些日光下无色，紫外光下有吸收的化合物也可应用。在腔内以稳定的流速通入氮气，可以防止流动相蒸发，同时可防止化合物氧化。

流动相洗脱时，化合物在薄层板上呈同心的圆形条带，最后又装在腔内的引管道处，用 TLC 检测洗脱流分。通常，50 ~ 500 mg（TLC R_f 0.2 ~ 0.5）混合物可用 2 mm 厚的板分离。开始洗脱时要用非极性的溶剂，接下来再慢慢增加极性。

4. 柱色谱　柱色谱是分离和纯化有机化合物的一种重要方法。它包括常压柱色谱、低压柱色谱、中压柱色谱和高压柱色谱。色谱材料包括硅胶、氧化铝、纤维素、聚酰胺、葡聚糖凝胶、活性炭、硅藻土等。柱色谱的洗脱剂通常为有机溶剂的混合或水和极性有机溶剂的混合物。硅胶柱色谱是经常使用的正相柱色谱，以有机溶剂的混合物为洗脱剂。而 C18 键合硅胶液相柱色谱是经常使用的反相柱色谱，以水和甲醇（或乙腈）的混合溶剂为洗脱剂。

扫码"看一看"

5. 重结晶　固体天然化合物达到一定的纯度，在一定的条件下，就会呈结晶状，这样就可以使结晶和母液分开，以达到进一步分离纯化的目的。有时结晶也是混合物，需要反复结晶，才能得到纯粹单一的结晶。

混合溶剂法重结晶，将粗晶溶于少量第一溶剂（使结晶易溶解的溶剂）中，然后加入恰好使溶液变成轻微混浊状所需要的足量溶剂。静置，冷至室温，结晶析出。同上操作收集晶体，必要时同法将产物进行第二次重结晶。详见实验一。

三、天然化合物的理化数据、波谱数据的测定与结构鉴定

1. 待测样品的纯度和干燥

（1）纯度　系统测定一个复杂化合物的结构，一般要求其纯度达到 95.0% ～ 100.0%。结构研究是天然药物化学的重要研究内容之一，在结构研究前必须测定化合物纯度，若纯度不合格，将给结构测定带来很大困难，甚至会导致结构测定的失败。例如，用 X 射线单晶衍射研究化合物结构时，对化合物的纯度要求非常高，一般需要大于 99.9%。

纯度鉴定的方法很多，如检查晶形、有无明确的熔点、熔距是否足够小等。但是最常用的还是各种色谱方法，如 TLC 或 PC 等。通常，只有当样品在三种不同的展开系统中呈现单一斑点时方可确认其为单体化合物。个别情况下，甚至必须采用正相和反相两种色谱方法加以确认。另外，气相色谱（GC）也是判断物质纯度的一种重要方法，但只适用于在高真空和一定加热条件下能够气化而不被分解的物质。HPLC 则不然，不受 GC 那样的条件限制。但却具有与 GC 一样，用量少、时间快、灵敏度高及准确的特点，但两者均需配置价格昂贵的仪器设备。很多情况下，纯化样品的目的就是为了波谱测定，以确定化合物的结构。

（2）样品的干燥　经提取、分离、纯化得到的化合物，需要进行干燥，然后再进行理化常数测定和结构鉴定，以进行深入研究。一方面，样品在干燥状态更加稳定；另外，计算得率及化合物结构确定均要求样品是干燥的。

①惰性气体下干燥　样品被干燥时，在样品表面和气相间形成动态平衡。通过带走样品表面的溶剂蒸气，平衡向溶剂蒸发的方向移动而达到干燥。这可以在加热或不加热条件下向样品通惰性气体如氮气来实现，最后在容器底部得到一层干燥的固体薄膜，但这种方法不易操作。

②旋转蒸发　旋转蒸发仪在大多数化学实验室都很常见，操作简单，在减压下使样品的沸点降低，旋转样品达到最大的表面积，溶剂蒸发。蒸气进入冷凝管，用另一容器收集，最后在圆底烧瓶内表面得到一薄层物质。

③真空干燥　常用干燥方法之一，原理是在真空装置中通过降低溶剂的沸点进行干燥，如果溶剂是水，一般在干燥器中加入干燥剂如五氧化二磷来吸水。如有必要，样品可加热。

④真空离心法　真空离心法具有低蒸气压和离心加热的双重优点，因此当样品被干燥后，样品集中在离心管底部而不是在一个较大的范围内分散成薄膜。这种方法适用于较大量液体样品的干燥，比如分析测定前的干燥和浓缩。

⑤冷冻干燥　这种方法的优点是，得到的样品具多孔结构，容易重新溶解或重新分散于溶液中。这种方法不会使蛋白质变性，也用于储存活的微生物细胞。

⑥其他　大多数情况下，物质在空气中干燥。可以在室温或不超过 30℃ 的烘箱中干燥；但必须远离阳光直射，因为紫外线可能引发化学反应生成人工产物。

2. 薄层色谱法　薄层色谱中的吸附剂是铺在玻璃、塑料或金属片或薄板上的较薄的、均匀的一层细粉状物质，因支持剂的种类、制备方法和选用溶剂的不同，可按吸附、分配或二者结合的方法达到分离化合物的目的。可以通过比较化合物的色谱行为，（如斑点的 R_f 值和显色情况）或将未知样品与对照品共薄层分析，对样品进行初步的鉴定。还可通过比

较可见斑点的大小进行半定量的判断，也可通过光密度测量法实现定量测定。

TLC 中涂布的物质与柱色谱用的吸附剂非常相似，如硅胶、氧化铝、聚酰胺等，只是它们的颗粒更细一些，一般直径为 5~40μm。有些还含有石膏、淀粉等黏合剂以增强涂层与薄板的黏合力。有些里面还含有荧光指示剂（如硅酸锌等），在 254nm 或 365nm 的紫外光下能显示荧光，可借此对分离的斑点进行检测。至今，硅胶仍然是最常用的薄层色谱吸附剂。

在涂布吸附剂时，用于排列和放置薄板的排列盘和具有平整表面的薄板是必需的。而涂布器也很常用，当它从玻璃板上移过时，会在板的表面均匀铺上所需厚度的吸附剂涂层。此外，也可手动铺板。

板铺好后，将要分析的几微升的样品溶液用毛细管点在板上，在板一侧点成小圆点，并使所有的点平行于板的一端呈直线排列。将板放到盛有少量溶剂的展开缸中。溶液通过毛细管作用带着样品组分沿着板展开。不同的组分因与吸附剂的相互作用程度差异而被分开。

（1）硅胶薄层色谱法 硅胶薄层色谱根据硅胶含水量的不同，可以是吸附色谱，也可以是分配色谱。

硅胶是至今薄层色谱中应用最多的一种固定相，多达 90% 的薄层分离都应用硅胶。硅胶为多孔性无定形粉末，表面带有硅醇基（silanol），呈弱酸性，通过硅醇基（吸附中心）与极性基团形成氢键而表现吸附性能，由于各组分的极性基团与硅醇基形成氢键的能力不同，使各组分被分离。硅胶吸附水分形成水合硅醇基而失去吸附能力，但加热后可被活化。

硅胶表面的 pH 约为 5，一般适合酸性和中性物质的分离，如有机酸、酚类、醛类等，这是因为碱性物质能与硅胶作用，展开时被吸附、拖尾，甚至停留在原点。

常用硅胶薄层色谱有硅胶 H、硅胶 G、硅胶 GF$_{254}$ 等。硅胶 H 为不含黏合剂的硅胶，铺成硬板时需另加黏合剂。硅胶 G 是硅胶和煅石膏混合而成。硅胶 GF$_{254}$ 除含煅石膏外另含有一种无机荧光剂，锰激活的硅酸锌，在 254 nm 紫外光下呈强烈黄绿色荧光背景。

（2）聚酰胺薄层色谱法 聚酰胺色谱属于氢键吸附色谱，是一种用途十分广泛的分离方法，极性物质与非极性物质均适用，特别适合于分离酚类，醌类及黄酮类化合物。

商品聚酰胺均为高分子聚合物，不溶于水、甲醇、乙醇、三氯甲烷及丙酮等有机溶剂，对碱较稳定，对酸尤其是无机酸稳定性较差，可溶于浓盐酸、冰醋酸及甲酸。

聚酰胺薄层色谱的常用展开剂是不同浓度的含水醇。此外，甲酰胺、二甲基甲酰胺及尿素水溶液也可作展开剂。在水中聚酰胺与酚类或醌类等化合物形成氢键缔合的能力最强，在含水醇中则随着醇浓度的增高而相应减弱，在高浓度醇或其他有机溶剂中则几乎不缔合。

聚酰胺的吸附强弱取决于各种化合物与聚酰胺形成氢键缔合的能力，在含水溶剂中大致有以下规律。

①形成氢键的基团数目越多，则吸附能力越强。

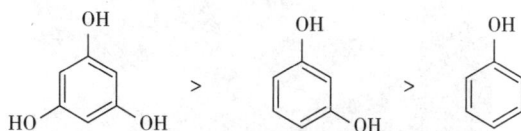

②易形成分子内氢键者，在聚酰胺上的吸附能力减弱。

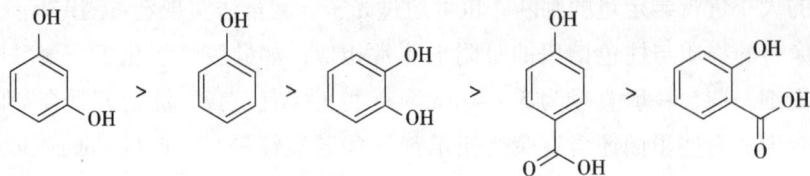

③分子中芳香化程度高者，吸附性增强。

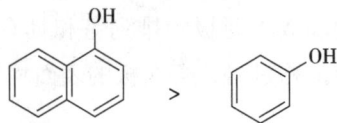

3. 纸色谱法　纸色谱法是以纸为载体的色谱法，其分离原理属于分配色谱。纸色谱过程可以看成是物质在固定相和流动相之间连续萃取的过程。根据物质在两相间分配系数的不同而达到分离的目的。与薄层色谱相同，纸色谱也常用比移值 R_f 来表示各组分在色谱中的位置。

通常，纸色谱属于正相分配色谱，化合物的极性大或亲水性强，在水中分配量多，则分配系数大，在以水为固定相的纸色谱中 R_f 值小；反之，则 R_f 值大。

纸色谱法的实验条件如下。

（1）色谱纸的选择　①要求滤纸质地均匀，应有一定的机械强度；②纸纤维的松紧适宜，过于疏松易使斑点扩散，过于紧密则流速过慢；③纸色应纯，无明显的荧光斑点。

（2）固定相　吸附在纤维素上的水为固定相，而纸纤维起到一个惰性载体的作用。

（3）展开剂　常用展开剂为含水的有机溶剂，如水饱和的正丁醇。为防止弱酸、弱碱的解离，加入少量的酸或碱，如甲酸、乙酸、吡啶等。

4. 熔点测定法　熔点测定是鉴定天然产物结晶纯度的方法之一。化合物的熔点有一个范围，在此范围内化合物由固相变成液相，这一过程有时伴随化合物的降解。纯的天然产物结晶一般都有一定的熔点和较小的熔距。当化合物中含有少量杂质会使实测熔点值降低。一些天然物有数个分解点或分解过程较长，有时不容易看清楚。有些则在加热过程中色泽逐渐变深，最后到分解，不易观察。有些立体异构体和同分异构体是结构非常类似的混合物，熔距也很短，还有些天然物有双熔点特性，即在某一温度已经全部熔化，当温度继续上升时又固化，然后在某一更高温度时又熔化或分解。双目镜熔点仪是一种常用的熔点测定仪（图1-6）。

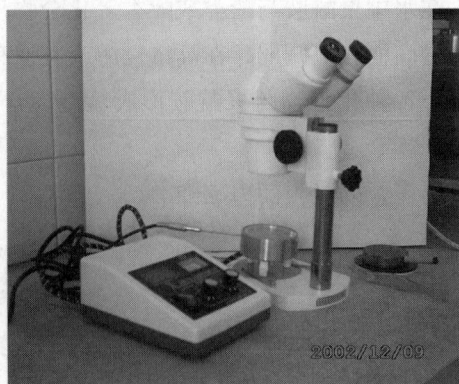

图1-6　双目镜熔点测定仪

5. 波谱法　现代有机化学中的结构鉴定主要依靠仪器方法，最常用的有：紫外－可见光谱、红外光谱、质谱及核磁共振光谱。

（1）紫外－可见吸收光谱（UV）　紫外－可见光谱是由于分子吸收紫外可见光由基态向激发态跃迁而引起的。用于检测共轭体系的电子跃迁并提供分子的共轭部分的长度和结构信息。紫外吸收的波长范围通常在 200～400 nm，对应的光子能量在 70～140 kcal/mol。若紫外吸收波长小于 200 nm，则其图谱很难处理，且也极少用于分析化合物的结构。

分子吸收紫外光的波长取决于分子轨道的电子能量，σ 键稳定而 π 键很容易吸收能量跃迁到较高能量的轨道。所以，在紫外－可见光范围内只有 n→π*，π→π* 跃迁可被观察，如图 1-7 所示。

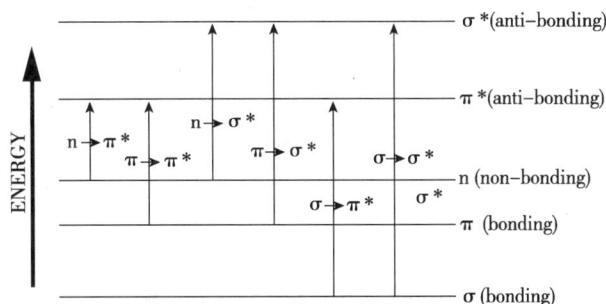

图 1-7　分子轨道电子跃迁能级图

大部分典型的紫外光谱吸收峰虽然比较宽，但用来判断分子中是否存在共轭 π 电子系统还是有用的。吸收最大处的波长用 λ$_{max}$ 表示。一个样品的吸收值 A 与溶液的浓度和紫外光束通过的液层厚度成正比。为校正溶度和液层厚度，将吸收值除以溶度 c（mol/L）和样品池的长度 l（cm），而转为摩尔吸收系数 ε。

$$\varepsilon = \frac{A}{c \cdot l}$$

摩尔吸收系数在 λ$_{max}$ 处测量，用 ε_{max} 表示，它通常没有单位。λ$_{max}$ 和 ε_{max} 受溶剂影响，所以在报道 UV-VIS 谱数据时要明确地标明溶剂的种类。

当有强吸收的生色团时，摩尔吸收系数可以非常大；而当吸收弱时，则非常小。

若一个化合物的紫外图谱中仅在 270～350 nm 区域有很弱的吸收带（ε = 10～100），且在 200 nm 以上无其他吸收，则该化合物含有一简单的非共轭生色团。

若一个化合物的紫外图谱中有多个吸收带，有些甚至出现在可见光范围内，则该化合物很有可能含有一长链的共轭结构或多芳香环生色团。若化合物有颜色，则至少含有 4～5 个共轭发色团或助色团。

ε 值在 10000 到 20000 之间代表化合物为 α，β 不饱和酮或二烯。

ε 值在 1000 到 10000 之间通常表示化合物中有一芳香系统。

用摩尔吸收系数的对数表示不饱和酮的紫外图谱更佳（图 1-8），242 nm 处的 π→π* 吸收很强，ε 为 18000；而 300 nm 附近的 n→π* 吸收则较弱，ε 仅为 100。

（2）红外吸收光谱（IR）　在核磁共振光谱出现以前，IR 是有机化合物结构鉴定中应用最多的仪器方法之一。虽然现在核磁共振光谱总的来说更能揭示一个未知化合物的结构，但 IR 在化学家所使用的光谱方法中仍保留着很重要的地位，因为它对鉴定分子中某些官能团的存在非常有用。

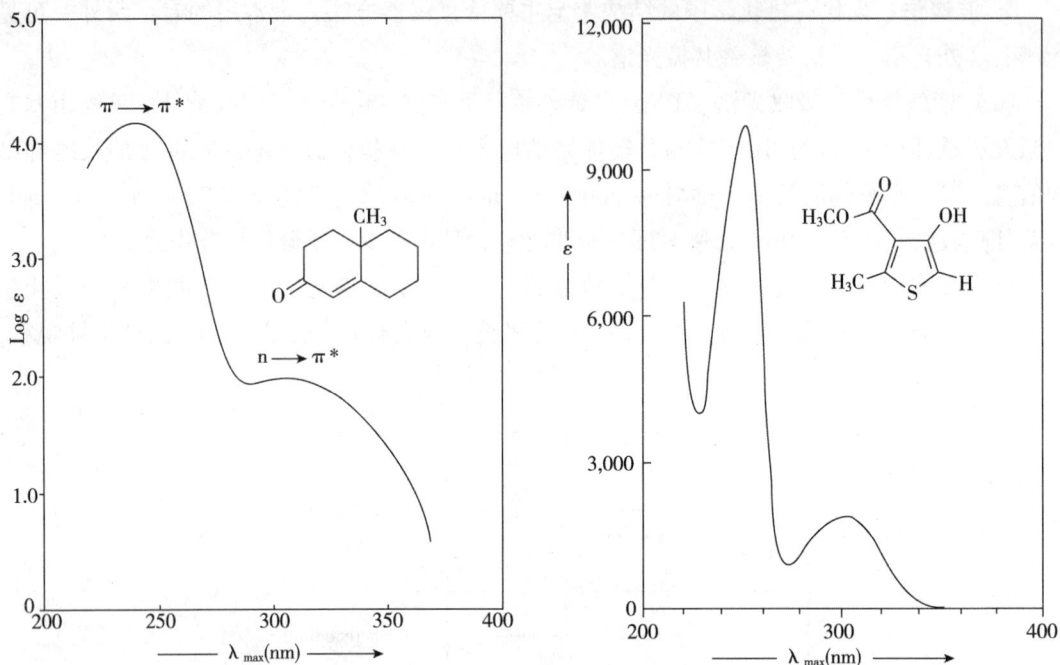

图 1-8 不饱和酮紫外波收图谱

IR 既可以用来获得化合物的结构信息，又可作为一种分析工具，测定化合物的纯度。其应用原理是基于这一事实：不同种类的官能团吸收不同波长的红外线。使用不同的样品池，红外光谱仪可检测气体、液体和固体等各种形态的样品。因此，在结构确定及化合物鉴定中，IR 是一种重要且常有的工具。

红外辐射位于电磁波谱中波长 14000 cm^{-1} 到 10 cm^{-1} 之间，而在这一区域内我们所关注的是中红外区（4000 ~ 400 cm^{-1}），因为其对应于分子的转动能级的跃迁；远红外区（400 ~ 10 cm^{-1}）在分析含有重原子的分子中非常有用，比如无机化学中的应用，但是需要专门的实验技术。

当化合物置于红外光束时，具有不同官能团的有机分子能吸收部分频率的红外射线，而其他频率的光则可以透过，所以红外谱图可以鉴定不同的官能团。

我们知道，分子有两种不同的振动形式：伸缩振动和弯曲振动。前者是沿着化学键的方向振动时键长有改变，包括对称伸缩振动和不对称伸缩振动；后者是引起键角变化的振动，包括剪式振动、面内摇摆、面外摇摆及面外弯曲振动。

IR 可分为两个不同的区域，一是特征区（4000 ~ 1500 cm^{-1}），该区域包含许多官能团的特征峰；另一区域为指纹区（1500 ~ 400 cm^{-1}），该区域非常复杂。但是，在指纹区内每种化合物都有自己的特征峰形，这可用于同系物的鉴定。不同类型化学键的红外伸缩频率见表 1-1。

表 1-1 不同类型化学键的红外伸缩频率

类型	波数 v（cm^{-1}）	强度
C≡N	2260 ~ 2220	中
C≡C	2260 ~ 2210	中
C═C	1690 ~ 1620	中到弱

类型	波数 ν（cm^{-1}）	强度
C—C	1680 ~ 1600	中
C≡N	1650 ~ 1550	中
⬡	1600 及 1500 ~ 1430	强到弱
C=O	1850 ~ 1650	强
C—O	1275 ~ 1050	强
C—N	1400 ~ 1020	中
O—H（醇）	3650 ~ 3200	强，宽
O—H（糖）	3300 ~ 2500	强，宽
N—H	3500 ~ 3100	中，宽
C—H	3300 ~ 2700	中

红外光谱测试常用仪器及测试方法如下。

1）傅里叶变换式红外光谱仪　当今，几乎所有的红外光谱仪都使用了傅里叶变换的方法，即在同一时间进行全波长扫描。这种方法有许多显而易见的优点：首先，该方法更快速，只用几秒而不是几分钟就可以记录一张完整的图谱；其次，该方法通过多层扫描及累加数据以增长信噪比，即使极少量或极稀的样品也可以得到一张完整的红外图谱。

2）样品的制备　依据被分析样品的物理性质，有不同的样品制备技术。

①固体样品　有两种制备样品的方法：石蜡糊法及 KBr 的压片法。

②液体样品　液体样品可用三明治法将其夹于两个高纯度的盐片之间（通常是氯化钠，溴化钾或氟化钙亦可）进行测定，盐片可透过红外光。

③气体样品　要得到气体样品的红外光谱，需要使用圆柱形气体槽，带有末端对红外不敏感的物质如 KBr、NaCl 或 CaF_2 组成的窗片，槽两端需封闭以便较容易的填充气体样品，进行红外分析测试。

（3）质谱（MS）　质谱是一种用来测定分子量的波谱方法，所用的样品量非常少，能给出分子量，对推导化合物的分子式很有价值，高分辨质谱能提供精确的分子式。

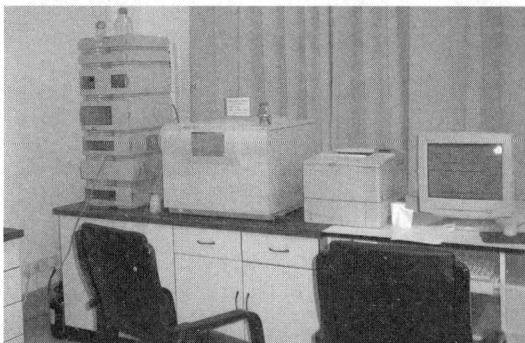

图 1 - 9　HP - 1100 型液 - 质联用仪

所有的质谱仪都需要将样品电离并且气化以便于分析，电离和气化可以同时发生，也可以分别进行。质谱仪（图 1 - 9）在高真空下把分子离子化，按照离子的质量分类，记录每个质量的离子丰度，然后即可绘出质谱图。

质谱仪常用的离子源包括电子电离（也称电子轰击）（EI）、化学电离（CI）、快原子轰击（FAB）、激光解析电离（MALDI）等，这里我们只讨论最常见的几种技术。

①电子轰击离子化（EI）　样品分子首先被气化，固体通常是插入一热探针，液体经过热隔膜和排气阀，气体经过一膜片和针型阀系统被气化。样品蒸气通过具有高能量（常为 70eV）的电子流，吸收其中的部分能量（通常在 20eV 左右），随之产生一系列电离过程。最简单的过程是样品分子通过失去一个电子而离子化，产生一正离子，为分子离子（$M^+ \cdot$），其质核比代表化合物的分子量。该方法最常用，但其缺点是（准）分子离子峰弱，将会影响分子量的测定；此外，样品分子必须能被气化，且在气化时必须是热稳定性的。

②化学电离法（CI）　首先，受电子轰击溶剂气体离子化，继而与样品分子反应而产生样品的离子，该方法可以给出分子量的相关信息但碎片离子较 EI 少。

③快原子轰击质谱（FAB）　该方法需要将样品溶解于基质（如甘油）中，因而样品必须附着在探针上。当样品表面用一高能的氙或氩原子轰击时，混合物将会溅射出离子，这些离子可能是正离子，也可能是负离子，每一种都能被分别检测到。

④基质辅助激光解析电离（MALDI）　该方法是基于固体试样放置于对光有吸收的基质中。通过高能量的激光照射样品，产生正负离子。

⑤高分辨质谱（HRMS）　高分辨质谱可用来确定化合物的分子式，用外加电场或磁场聚焦形成精确的电磁束，检测粒子质量，可精确到 1/20000，HRMS 能够提供准确的化合物相对分子质量，由此可确定化合物的准确分子式。

（4）核磁共振波谱（NMR）　在过去的 50 年里，核磁共振波谱已成为测定有机化合物结构的非常有效的工具。同 IR 一样，NMR 用量少，对样品无破坏。许多化合物的结构仅用 NMR 就可推断，而测定很多复杂化合物的结构，则需与其他方法相结合（图 1 – 10）。

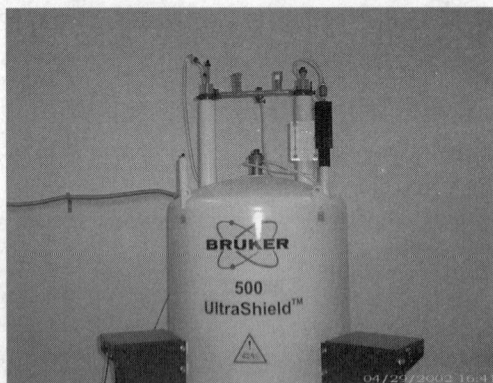

图 1 – 10　500MHz 核磁共振仪

原则上，核磁共振适用于任何具有自旋的核。天然存在的同位素核都有其特征自旋，一些自旋为整数（$I = 1, 2, 3, \cdots$），另外一些为半整数（$I = 1/2, 3/2, 5/2, \cdots$），还有一些没有自旋，$I = 0$。在有机化学中，最重要的是 $I = 1/2$ 的核，包括 ^1H、^{13}C、^{19}F 和 ^{31}P。对于有机化学家来讲，最重要的是核磁共振氢谱（^1H–NMR）和核磁共振碳谱（^{13}C–NMR）。

我们知道核的自旋有 $2I + 1$ 种可能的取向，所以在外加磁场中 $I = 1/2$ 的核将有两种自旋状态，这两种自旋状态能量差别很小，并且取决于外加磁场的强度。当外加磁场强度为零时，这两种状态的自旋核有相同的能量；当外加磁场强度不为零时，则两种核的能量亦不同（图1-11）。

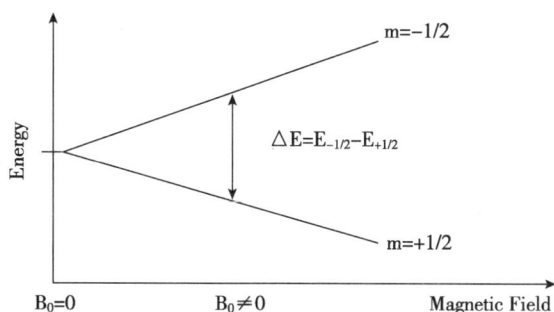

图1-11　在外加磁场中 I=1/2 的核的两种自旋状态能量差

^{1}H-NMR 能够提供给我们的信息有化学位移和自旋-自旋偶合。

①化学位移（δ）　化学家将有机分子中的氢原子化学位移与一种标准物质中的氢相比，并以此来比较该分子中的氢所受的屏蔽。这种标准物质就是四甲基硅烷，$(CH_3)_4Si$，简写为 TMS。化学位移常用 δ 表示（ppm）。例如，乙醇（CH_3CH_2OH）的 ^{1}H-NMR 中，有对应于三个特征化学位移处的三组特征信号，分别为甲基信号、亚甲基信号及羟基信号。甲基特征峰化学位移为 1 ppm，与羟基相连的亚甲基化学位移约为 4 ppm，而羟基因所用溶剂不同在 2~3 ppm 之间。峰的形状与大小也是鉴定化合物结构的指标，如上例中的乙醇谱图中，甲基峰是羟基峰的三倍。同样，亚甲基峰是羟基峰的二倍，但仅为甲基峰的 2/3。常见质子的化学位移见图 1-12。

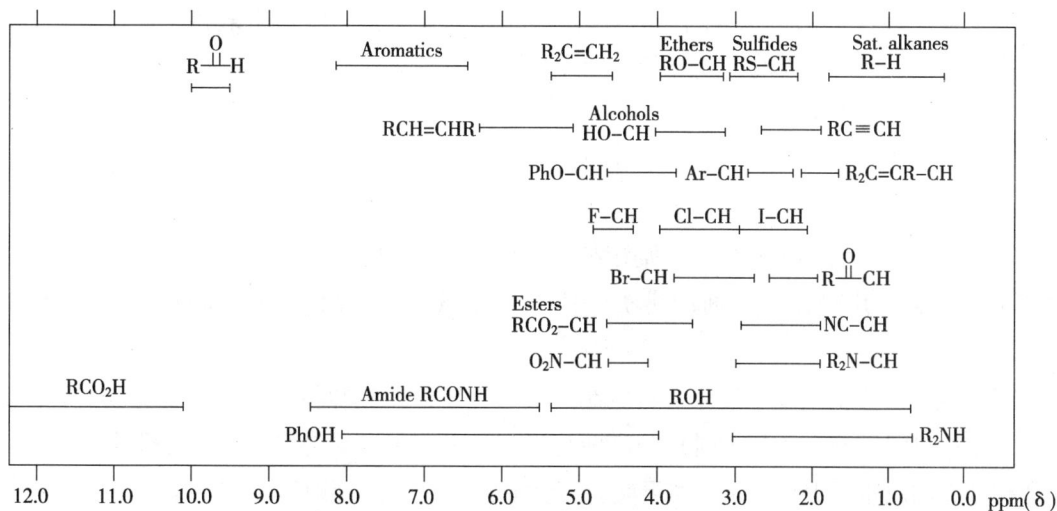

图1-12　常见质子的化学位移

②自旋-自旋偶合　我们知道，处于相同化学环境或化学位移的核是等价的，而那些在不同化学环境或化学位移下的核是不等价的。相互临近的核会对彼此的有效磁场产生影响。反映在 NMR 谱中，就是化学不等价核会产生很多组峰。这种效应称之为自旋-自旋耦合。这种耦合可提供详细的信息来分析分子中原子间的连接关系。判断核磁共振谱中质子裂分的一般规律：裂分的峰数为 n+1 个，n 代表相邻的等价质子数：无邻位质子，为单峰（s）；一个邻位质子，为双峰（d）；两个邻位质子，为三重峰（t）；三个邻位质子，为四重峰

（q）等。例如，上面提及的乙醇氢谱图中，甲基质子受邻位亚甲基质子的偶合，裂分为强度比为 1：2：1 的三重峰；类似的，亚甲基质子受邻位甲基质子的偶合，裂分为强度比为 1：3：3：1 的四重峰。

四、设计性实验的设计思路和实施方法

以下具体内容均以补骨脂素和异补骨脂素的提取分离和鉴定为例。

1. 药材来源　补骨脂为豆科补骨脂属植物补骨脂（*Psoralea corylifolia* L.）的种子，为温肾壮阳、纳气、止泻药。用于阳痿遗精、遗尿、尿频、腰膝冷痛、肾虚作喘。补骨脂中主要含有补骨脂素、异补骨脂素和黄酮类化合物。

2. 实验目的

（1）学习查阅天然药物化学主要国内外文献的方法。

（2）学习整理文献资料、撰写综述的方法。

（3）通过分析文献资料，综合所学知识，自行设计并实施提取分离补骨脂素和异补骨脂素的方法；并将分离得到的单体成分进行结构鉴定。

（4）学习并初步掌握香豆素类化合物的提取分离和结构鉴定方法。

3. 实验安排

（1）查阅文献，撰写综述

外文文献：检索 Scifinder，CA 光盘数据库，Medline 光盘数据库等。

中文文献：检索中国药学光盘数据库、中国生物医学数据库等。

要求学会系统查阅国内外文献的方法，有详细的查阅记录及资料，撰写综述，其内容包括：①补骨脂的植物来源、品种、科属及分布；②补骨脂、补骨脂素和异补骨脂素的临床应用和药理活性研究概况；③补骨脂中主要化合物的名称、熔点、结构、理化性质、提取分离及结构鉴定方法。

（2）文献交流，设计实验方案　要求对已经撰写的文献进行充分的交流和讨论，在此基础上，以组为单位设计实验方案，其主要内容包括：①提取方法，所用提取装置，提取溶剂的种类及用量；②纯化方法，所用装置，使用的溶剂及用量；③分离方法，选用的色谱填料的种类、用量，洗脱剂的种类、比例及用量；④列出所需实验材料，安排实验进度。

（3）实验方案的实施　按照自行定制的实验方案，在教师指导下，独立完成实验，要求在规定的时间周期内（如 3 周）分离纯化得到补骨脂素和异补骨脂素单体化合物，每一单体化合物的质量不少于 5mg。如果实验方案有所调整，应及时通知指导老师，以便提供必要的实验材料，保证实验顺利进行。

将分离得到的单体化合物进行理化性质以及必须的波谱数据的测定。

（4）实验结果讨论　每组先自行整理实验记录，讨论实验结果，总结实验得失。再进行全班集中讨论，检查实验产品的质量，交流实验操作的经验，比较不同实验方案的优劣。

（5）完成实验报告　对本组实验全过程进行总结讨论，提出本组实验成功与失败之处，评价不同实验方案的优劣，提出可改进之处，完成实验报告。

Part I Common Experimental Methods in Natural Pharmaceutical Chemistry

I. Extration

1. Extraction

The purpose of extraction and isolation are separating the desired compounds from the other components by all means. There are numerous complex compounds in plants, some of them are considered having good activities, such as alkaloids, terpenes, steroids, flavones, anthraquinones, coumarins, organic acids, amino acids, monosaccharides, oligosaccharides, polysaccharides, proteins, enzymes, tannins and so on. Whereas others like celluloses, chlorophylls, waxes, greases, resins and gums, are thought as ineffective substances and often threw away in our research. The following is about some methods that are frequently used during extraction and separation.

1.1 Water – extraction

Water – extraction was achieved in three ways: decocting, immersing and percolation, acid and alkali sometimes are used to promote the extract efficiency for acidic and alkalic compounds. Some natural acids, alkalis, glycosides, and small molecule (for example, berberine, glycyrrhizinic acid and globulariacitrin) can dissolve in water, so water was often chosen as extracting solvent. But, water may dissolve many substances that (eg. inorganic salts, proteins, saccharides and starches) are adverse to further separation. Therefore, some compounds are extracted by organic solvents in order to bring out less useless components, although they are dissolvable in water.

1.2 Organic solvent-extraction

Organic solvent-extraction often carry out with reflux extraction, soxhlet extraction, immersing and percolation. Several solvents in different polarity may be used from low polarity to high polarity. Different solubility of each component under different polarity realize the separation. Single solvent may also be used. Ethanol has good dissolution ability and strong penetration power. So ethanol-water in different ratios is the best choice of single solvent. The concentration is decided by the characteristic of extracted components.

1.3 Water vapor distillation

Volatile oil and some volatile components are able to be separated by water vapor distillation. For example, efedrina is separated directly from Ephedra by this method.

2. Filtration

Filtration is a simple method to separate solid from liquid. It is often used to eliminate insoluble materials in solutions and remove drug residues when extraction finished. In general, filtration is realized by filter papers and funnels, sometimes column filtration is also adopted.

3. Concentrate

Concentration of extract can usually carry out by rotary evaporation and freeze drying. Rotary

13

evaporators are familiar to most chemical laboratories. The process is simply boiling the sample under a reduced pressure to lower the boiling point while rotating the sample to maximize the surface area when evaporation takes place. The vapor is condensed by a condenser and collected in a separated vessel. The material may end up as a thin film across the inside of the glass round-bottomed flask. During rotary evaporation, solution containing surface-active material is prone to frothing forming a foam that can spill out of the containing vessel. This can sometimes be reduced by the addition of a small amount of surface-active organic solvent such as n-butanol. Freeze-drying takes place under high vacuum and involves sublimation of water from a frozen solid. The sample to be dried is first frozen, using solid carbon dioxide. Then place the sample under vacuum and the water removed by sublimation. When the sample undergoing a drying step ceases to lose weight, it has no more solvent left to lose and is therefore dry.

II. Several methods in separation and purification

1. Extraction

The most frequently used extraction method is liquid-liquid distribution extraction. Different distribution coefficients of compounds in two solvents that is immiscible make themselves separated. When water or alcohol system is used as extraction solutions, evaporating the extract into dense water solution. Then extracting the solution with suitable organic solvent. If the desire materials are liposoluble, the organic solvents choices can be petroleum ether, chloroform or diethylether. If the materials are hydrophilic, ethyl acetate and butanol can be chosen.

2. Desalting and removal of chlorophyll

2.1 Desalting

Desalting is probably one of the most important step in the handling of water-solube compounds. It is not necessarily difficult to fractionate water-solube compounds. This is the step in which organic chemists may simple partition between water-immiscible organic solvents and aqueous solutions.

If the effective compounds have some lipophicity, the standard method for desalting is the use of reverse phase columns such as C18 silica gel or various other organic polymers such as XAD-2, -4, and-7. Usually, the as aqueous solution is passed through the column and salts are washed out with water; subsequently, the effective compounds are eluted with a solvent system containing organic solvents. This method cannot be applied to strongly polar or ionized compounds such as polar amino acids or sugars. Another commonly used method for desalting is the use of size-exclusion columns such as Sephadex G-10 and Bio-Gel P-2. Because of the unpredictive interection of inorganic ions, compounds and column supports, the predicted elution order can often be reversed. These interactions can hold advantages for the extractor and can be used to isolate specific types of compounds.

In most cases, it is necessary to use the buffer solutions in the extraction and fraction of water-soluble compounds. In other words, the key to the isolation of water-soluble compounds is finding a suitable pH and ionic concentration to keep the molecules as individual molecular entities separable on a given matrix. However, the separation of the buffers salts from the compound is not an easy task. They are mostly combinations of weak bases and weak acids, which are bound only by weak ionic interactions and are volatile under reduced pressure or lyophilization. However, in reality, these buffers are not so easy to handle.

2. 2 Remove of chlorophyll

Chlorophyll, a kind of green pigmen, exists widely in plants, especially in leaves. It is dissolvable in general organic solvents, and nearly undissolvable in water. Chlorophyll in water extracts can be removed by extracting with petroleum ether or chloroform. Adding water to ethanol extracts or evaporating ethanol from ethanol-water solvent until the concentration become 15% ~ 20% and then refrigerating, chlorophyll will be precipitated. In addition, chlorophyll is dissolvable in basic water, but insoluble in water. Because of that characteristic, chlorophyll also can be removed by acid and base treatment, but the desired material must be resistant and dissolves in water or don't dissolve in basic water.

3. Centrifugal thin-layer chromatography

Classical preparative thin-layer chromatography has several drawbacks. The main disadvantage is mixing with inpyrities when the target compound was taken off the plate and eluting adsorbent in the subsequent extraction. Other drawbacks include the too length time required for a separation and the presence of impurities and residues from the plate itself, found after solvent extraction of the zones containing the product.

In order to overcome some of these problems, a number of approaches involving centrifugal chromatography have been attempted. The technique of centrifugal chromatography is, in principle, classical TLC with an accelerated flow of mobile phase produced by the action of a centrifugal force: a forced flow method.

The big difference between the Chromatofuge and its predecessors lies in the fact that the rotor is inclined rather than horizontal. The heart of the apparatus is a 24cm diameter circular glass plate which is covered with a suitable sorbent, to provide the thin layer for preparative separations. In order to prevent breaking up of the thin layer, the sorbent is mixed with a binder. For the majority of separations on silica gel, the sorbent is mixed with a binder. For the majority of separations on silica gel, the following recipe for a single 2mm plate can be used. Silica gel GF_{254} for TLC （60g） is mixed with 0. 8% CMC-Na （180ml） in a 250ml Erlenmeyer flask. Water （110ml） is added and vigorously shaken for 30s. The slurry is poured onto the plate and made spread out into a relatively uniform layer. Overnight drying at room temperature is followed oven heating at 60 ~ 70℃. After cooling, the surface of the sorbent is smoothed by scraping tool fixed to the centre of the plate. A small area is left free in the middle to allow introduction of eluent. Other recipes for the preparation of plates include silica gel plates with silver nitrate, and aluminum oxide. Binding reversed phase material to the glass plates is a much more difficult task.

The prepared plate （1, 2 or 4 mm sorbent thickness） is screwed onto the hub of an electric motor and rotated at 800 rpm. Eluent is introduced onto the sorbent-free centre of the plate via a piston pump capable of delivering 1 ~ 10ml/min, and passes across the thin layer under the influence of the centrifugal force. The rotor is first washed for several minutes to remove impurities present in the adsorbent. Following this step, two options are available. Elution is then continued, either with a solvent of constant composition or with a step gradient, at $3 \sim 6$ ml/min.

The rotor until is housed in a chamber covered with a quartz glass plate. This cover enables the observation of colourless but UV-active substance zones with the aid of o UV lamp. A steady flow of nitrogen is passed though the chamber to prevent evaporation of the eluent and to avoid oxidation of the sample. Introduction of sample, followed by solvent elution gives concentric bands of the components. At the periphery, the bands are spun off and collected through an exit tube in the chamber. Fractions of eluate thus obtained are analysed by TLC. In general, $50 \sim 500$ mg of a mixture can be separated on a 2mm layer, as long as the R_f on an analytical TLC plate lies between 0.2 and 0.5. Weakly polar solvent systems should be used at the beginning of the separation, with a gradual increase in polarity during the run.

4. Colum chromatography

Column chromatography (CC) is an important method for the separation and purification of organic compounds, including normal phase LCC and reverse phase LCC, as well as normalpreswsure, low preswsure, moderate pressure and high pressure LCC. The packing material of the columns include silica gel, alumina oxide, cellulose, polyamide, sephadex, activated carbon, celite and so on. The eluting solvents or mobile phases for LCC are usually mixtures of organic solvents (e. g. methanol, or/and acetonitrile). Silica LCC is often used as normal phase LCC, using mixtures of organic solvents as eluting solvents. And C-18 bonded silica gel LCC is often used as reverse phase LCC, using mixtures of water and methanol or acetonitrile as eluting solvents.

5. Recrystallization

When solid natural compounds reach to a certain purity, under certain condition, it was crystal. So it can realize the separation of crystallization from mother liquor in order to achieve the purpose of further separation and purification. Sometimes crystallization is a mixture, so recrystallization need to be repeatedly carried on in order to obtain pure single crystal.

Mixed solvent recrystallization: we dissolve coarse crystalline in a small amount of the first solvent (in which the crystallization dissolves eaaily), and then add adequate solvent (in which the cryatallization is insoluble) to make the solution become slightly turbid. Standing, cooling to room temperature, cryatallization. For details, see Experiment I.

III. The physical and chemical information, spectra data, and structure determination of natural compounds

1. The purity and drying of samples

1.1 Purify

To assign a complex structure, the $95\% \sim 100\%$ purity of a compound is generally required. The structure research is one of the most important parts in natural product chemistry. Prior to structure research, it must first determine the purity of compounds. Unqualified purity will lead to greater difficulty of the work, and may even lead to the failure of the work of structure determination.

For example, in X-ray crystallography studies, material will be required in an extremely pure state, generally >99.9% pure. On the other hand, if a natural product is required for biological testing, it is important to know the degree of purity and the nature of the impurities. If a compound is to be used to generate pharmacological or pharmacokinetic data, it is usually important that the material be very pure (generally > 99% pure) .

There are many ways to check the purity of compounds, such as checking for the crystal shape, with or without a clear and sharp melting point and so on. However, the most commonly used is a variety of chromatography methods, such as TLC or PC. Generally, only when the sample in three different solvent systems show a single spot, can be regarded as a single compound. In individual circumstances, it may require the use of normal phase and reverse phase chromatography to confirm the two. In addition, gas chromatography (GC) used to determine the material purity is an important method, but apply only to materials which are stable at high vacuum and heating conditions. HPLC will not need the same conditions as GC. Like with GC, but also less used, time fast, sensitive and accurate, but they all require the expensive equipment. In many cases, the aim of the purification will be to carry out spectroscopy in order to elucidate molecular structure.

1. 2 Drying

After separation, extraction and purification, compounds should be dried and then proceed to the determination of physical and chemical constants and structural identification for the further work of composition. The compound is more likely to remain stable in a dry form. In order to determine the yield of isolated, it usually needs to be weighed as a dry solid.

1. 2. 1 Drying under inert gas

As a sample is dried, a dynamic equilibrium is established between the sample surface and the vapor phase. By removing solvent vapor from the immediate vicinity of the surface, the equilibrium is shifted in favor of evaporation and drying. This can be done by passing an insert gas such as nitrogen over a sample either with or without additional heating. This method may leave the solid as a dry film on the bottom of the vessel, but not always easy to manipulate.

1. 2. 2 Rotary evaporation

Rotary evaporators are familiar to most chemical laboratories, and the process is simply one of boiling the sample under a reduced pressure to lower the boiling point while rotating the sample to maximize the surface area over which evaporation takes place. The vapor is trapped by a condenser and collects in a separate vessel. Again the material may end up as a thin film across the inside of a glass round-bottomed flask. An additional disadvantage is that solutions may be prone to " bump" , or boil unevenly, spilling over into the waste vessel.

1. 2. 3 Vacuum drying

Usually we dry materials in this method. This process essentially follows the principle with an applied vacuum facilitating drying by lowering the boiling point of the solvent. If the solvent is water, a hygroscopic material such as phosphorus pentoxide is normally put in the dryer to absorb water. The sample can be heated as necessary.

1. 2. 4 Vacuum centrifugation

Vacuum centrifugation combines the advantages of low vapor pressure and heating with centrifugation, so that as samples dry, they are concentrated in the bottom of a tube rather than spread as a thin film over a relatively large area. This method is particularly useful for handling relatively large numbers of liquid samples such as drying and concentrating fractions prior to assay.

1.2.5 Freeze-drying

Freeze-drying takes place under high vacuum and involves sublimation water from a frozen solid. The sample to be dried is first frozen, using solid carbon dioxide or freon, and placed under vacuum and the water removed by sublimation. This process has the advantage that it tends to leave the sample as a manageable solid with a fine porous structure that allows it to be readily redissolved or resuspended in liquid. It tends not to denature proteins and can be used as a means of storing viable microbial cells.

1.2.6 Others

In most cases, plant material is dried in the atmosphere. It may be dried at room temperature or in the oven at no more than 30℃, and it must be kept away from direct sunlight because ultraviolet radiation may produce chemical reactions giving rise to compound artifacts.

2. Thin-layer chromatography (TLC)

In thin-layer chromatography, the adsorbent is a relatively thin, uniform layer of finely powered material applied to a glass, plastic, or mental sheet or plate, glass plates being commonly employed. The separations achieved may be based upon adsorption, partition, or a combination of both effects, depending on the particular type of support, its preparation, and its use with different solvents.

Presumptive identification can be effected by observation of spot of identical R_f value and about equal magnitude obtained, respectively, with an unknown and a reference sample chromatography on the same plate. A visual comparison of the spots may serve for semi quantitative analysis. Quantitative measurements are possible by means of densitometry.

The coating materials of TLC are similar to the sorbents used for column chromatography except that are generally of a smaller particle size, such as silica, alumina, polyamide etc. , normally $5 \sim 40$ μm in diameter. Some of those contain a binder such as plaster of Paris ($CaSO_4$) or starch to adherence of the film to the plate. An insert fluorescent indicator (e. g. Zinc silicate) which fluoresces when illuminated with 254 or 365 UV light so as to aid in the detection of separated spots is also sometimes including. Silica is by far the most used adsorbent for TLC.

An aligning tray and a flat surface upon must be employed which to align and rest the plates during the application of the adsorbent. A spreader is always used also, which will apply a uniform layer of adsorbent of desired thickness over the entire surface of the plate, when move over the glass plate. The plate can also be made by hand.

When the plate was made, a few micro-liters of a solution of the sample to be analyzed are spotted onto the plate as a single small dot near one end of the plate using a micro-capillary tube. Be sure that all mixture spots are lined up parallel to the edge of the plate. The plate is developed by placing it in a jar or developing chamber that contains a small amount of solvent. The solvent rises up to the plate by capillary action, carrying the components of the sample with it. The different compounds are separated based upon their interaction with the adsorbent coating.

2.1 Silica TLC

The stationary phase of silica TLC gel is silica gel. According to the different water content, either adsorption chromatography or partition chromatography can also be. Silica is by far the most used adsorbent for TLC, about a maximum of 90% of the silica gel thin-layer separation are applied. As porous and amorphous powder, there is silanol on gel surface which show weak acid. The formation of hydrogen-bond between silicon (adsorption center) and the polar groups shows adsorption properties. Since the ability of the different components to form hydrogen-bond with silanol is different, various components are separated. Silica gel adsorbing water will lose absorbability because of losing silanol. However, this can be activated after heating.

The pH on silica surface is about 5, which is suitable to separate acid and neutral materials, such as organic acids, phenols, aldehydes and so on. Because of an alkaline substance having a role with the silica gel, it may be carried out adsorption, tailing, and even stay fixed at the origin.

The commonly used silica gel in thin-layer chromatography is silica gel H, silica gel G and silicagel GF_{254} and so on. Silica gel H is the non-adhesive silicone gel, adding plus when paving hard board. Silica G is a mixture of dried gypsum and silica gel, while silica gel GF_{254} containing an inorganic fluorescent agent which shows a strong yellow-green fluorescence background under ultra-violet light in the 254nm.

2.2 Polyamide TLC

Polyamide adsorption, based on hydrogen bond, is a very broad use of methods of separation. Both polar substances and non-polar substances can be applied, particularly suitable for separation of phenols, quinones, and flavonoids.

Commercial polyamide is polymers of giant molecule, which are not soluble in water, methanol, ethanol, chloroform, acetone and other organic solvents. It's more stable in base, but not stable in acid, especially in inorganic acid. It can dissolve in concentrated hydrochloric acid, glacial acetic acid and formid acid.

The commonly used developing solvent of polyamide thin-layer chromatography is different concentrations of alcohol. In addition, formamide, dimethyl formamide and aqueous solution of urea can also be used as developing solvents. The ability to form hydrogen bond between polyamide and phenolic compounds or quinones is the strongest in the water. Along with the concentration of alcohol increased, the association ability decline corresponding. It's almost non-association in concentrated alcohol or other organic agents.

The adsorption strength of polyamide depends on the ability of a variety of compounds and polyamide to form hydrogen bonds. There are laws as follows in the aqueous solution.

2.2.1 The more hydrogen bonds formation, the stronger the adsorption capacity.

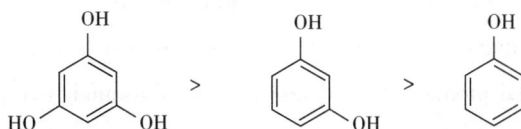

2.2.2 The easier to form intra-molecular hydrogen bonds, the weaker to adsorb to polyamide.

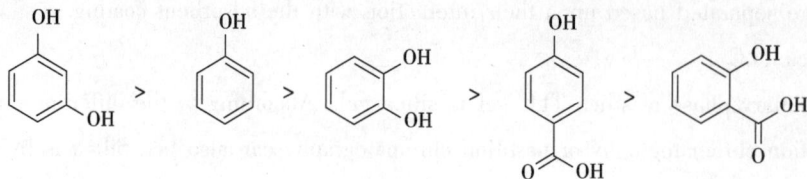

2. 2. 3 The adsorption ability increased if molecules with a high degree of aromatization.

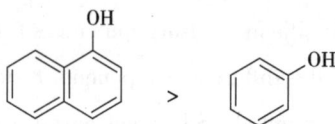

3. Paper chromatography

Paper chromatography, which the carrier is paper, is a kind of chromatography with the separation principle is partition. The process of paper chromatography can be regarded as the continuous extraction process of solute in two phases, we can achieve separation purpose. As the same as thin-layer chromatography, retardation factor is also used to indicate the location of each component in chromatography.

Generally, paper chromatography is normal phase partition chromatography. For polar compounds or hydrophilic materials, the distribution volume in the water is large, so as to the distribution coefficient and R_f value is small in the water as the stationary phase in paper chromatography with water as the stationary phase. Conversely, the R_f is large.

The experimental conditions of paper chromatography。

3. 1 The choice of paper　①Uniform quality of filter paper is required and there should be a certain degree of mechanical strength. ②The elastic fibers are suitable for paper. If fiber is too loose, the spot is easy to spread. If too tight, it will flow slowly. ③Paper color should be pure without any significant fluorescence spots.

3. 2 Stationary phase　The water adsorbed in thionary phase, and the paper fibers play the role of an inert carrier.

3. 3 Developing solvent　The most commonly used developing solvent in paper chromatography is water-bearing organic solvents, such as water-saturated n-butanol. In order to prevent weak acid or weak base dissociation, by adding a small amount of acid or alkali, such as formic acid, acetic acid, and pyridine and so on.

4. Melting point determination

Melting point determination is one of the methods to detect the purity of crystal of natural product. The melting point of compounds is a broad range, which in this course the compound changed from the solid phase into liquid phase and sometimes accompanied by the degradation of compounds. Pure natural crystalline compound has a certain melting point and a narrow melting-point range. Compounds containing a small amount of impurities will lower the value of the measured melting point. Some natural products have decomposition of a number of points or a longer distance of decomposition and sometimes it is not easy to see. Some become darker in color gradually in the process of heating. Finally, the contraction point is not clear until the compound is decomposed.

The melting-point range of some stereoisomer and structural isomer which are very similar to a mixture is also narrow. Some natural products have a double melting point, that is, they have all been melted in a melting temperature, become solid when the temperature continuous to rise, and then at a higher temperature they are melting or decomposing. Double binocular microscope melting point determination apparatus is a commonly used detector.

5. Spectrum analysis

The task of structure determination in modern-day organic chemistry relies heavily on instrumental methods. The most generally used methods are: Ultraviolet-visible spectroscopy (UV), Infrared spectroscopy (IR), Mass spectrometry (MS) and Nuclear magnetic resonance spectroscopy (NMR).

5. 1 Ultraviolet / Visible spectroscopy

We know ultraviolet/ visible spectroscopy (UV) involves the absorption of ultraviolet/ visible light by a molecule causing the promotion of an electron from a ground electronic state to an excited electronic state. Ultraviolet (UV) spectroscopy detects the electronic transitions of conjugated systems and provides information about length and structure of the conjugated part of the molecule. UV spectroscopy gives more specialized information than do IR or NMR, and it less commonly used than the other techniques. Ultraviolet radiation have wavelengths between 200 to 400nm (2×10^{-5} to 4×10^{-5} cm), corresponding to photon energies of about 70 to 140 kcal/mol. If ultraviolet radiation having wavelengths less than 200nm is difficult to handle, and is seldom used as a routine tool for structural analysis.

The wavelengths of UV light which a molecule absorbed are determined by the electronic energy difference between orbitals in the molecule. Sigma bonds are stable while Pi bonds are easily excited into higher energy orbitals. So only the two lowest energy ones are achieved by the energies available in the 200 to 400nm spectrum.

As is typical of most UV spectra, the absorption peak is rather broad but sometimes useful in indicating the presence of particular conjugated π-electron systems within a molecule. The wavelength at which absorption is a maximum is referred to as the λmax of the sample. The absorbance A of a sample is proportional to its concentration in solution and the path length through which the beam of ultraviolet radiation passes. To correct for concentration and path length, absorbance is converted to molar absorptivity ε by dividing it by the concentration c in moles per liter and the path length in centimeters.

$$\varepsilon = \frac{A}{c \cdot l}$$

Molar absorptivity, when measured at λ_{max}, is cited as ε_{max}. It is normally expressed without units. Both λ_{max} and ε_{max} are affected by the solvent, so it is explicitly indicated when reporting UV-VIS spectroscopic data.

Molar absorptivities may be very large for strongly absorbing chromophores (> 10000) and very small if absorption is weak (10 to 100).

If the spectrum of a given compound exhibits an absorption band of very low intensity (e = 10 ~ 100) in the 270 ~ 350nm region, and no other absorptions above 200nm, the compound contains a simple, nonconjugated chromophore.

If the spectrum of a given compound exhibits many bands, some of which appear even in the visible region, the compound is likely to contain long-chain conjugated or polycyclic aromatic chromophore. If the compound is colored, there may be at least 4 to 5 conjugated chromophores and auxochromes.

A ε value between 10000 and 20000 generally represents a simple α, β-unsaturated ketone or diene.

Bands with ε values between 1000 and 10000 normally show the presence of an aromatic system.

A few examples are displayed below. The spectrum of the unsaturated ketone illustrates the advantage of a logarithmic display of molar absorptivity. The $\pi \rightarrow \pi^*$ absorption located at 242nm is very strong, with an $\varepsilon = 18000$. The weak $n \rightarrow \pi^*$ absorption near 300nm has an $\varepsilon = 100$。

5.2 Infrared spectroscopy (IR)

Prior to the introduction of NMR spectroscopy, infrared (IR) spectroscopy was the instrumental method most often applied to structure determination of organic compounds. While NMR spectroscopy is, in general, more revealing of the structure of an unknown compound, IR still retains an important place in the chemists inventory of spectroscopic methods because of its usefulness in identifying the presence of certain functional groups within a molecule.

Infrared spectroscopy, referred to as IR which is commonly used both to gather information about the structure of a compound and as an analytical tool to assess the purity of a compound. It is based on the fact that different chemical functional groups absorb infrared light at different wavelengths dependent upon the nature of the particular chemical function group. Using various sampling accessories. IR spectroscopy is an important and popular tool for structural elucidation and compound identification.

The infrared region of the electromagnetic spectrum extends from 14000cm^{-1} to 10cm^{-1}. The region which we interest is the mid-infrared region (4000cm^{-1} to 400cm^{-1}), which corresponds to changes in irrational energies within molecules. The far infrared region (400cm^{-1} to 10cm^{-1}) is useful for molecules containing heavy atoms such as inorganic compounds but requires rather specialized experimental techniques.

When compounds positioned in the path of an IR beam, some frequencies of IR radiation are absorbed by the compounds which have different functional groups while others passed. So the IR spectrum can identify the different functional groups.

We know that there are two different types of molecular vibrations, stretching and bending. The former is a vibration along the bond that changes the bond length, which contains two types, symmetric stretch and asymmetric stretch. The later is a vibration that changes the bond angle. Four types of this bond: rocking, scissoring, wagging and twisting.

The infrared spectrum: IR spectrum can be divided into two different areas, one is functional group region ($4000 \sim 1500\ \text{cm}^{-1}$), which contains many of the functional groups that showed absorption bands. The other is fingerprint region ($1500 \sim 400\text{cm}^{-1}$) which is quite complex in this region. In this area many compounds have characteristic spectrum, which can be used to identify homologues. Here the IR stretching frequencies associated with different types of bonds are show in the Table 1 – 1.

Table　1 – 1　Stretching frequencies associated with different typer of bonds

Type of Bond	Wavenumber, ν (cm^{-1})	intensity
C≡N	2260 ~ 2220	medium
C≡C	2260 ~ 2210	medium
C=C	1690 ~ 1620	medium to weak
C—C	1680 ~ 1600	medium
C≡N	1650 ~ 1550	medium
⬡	1600 and 1500 ~ 1430	strong to weak
C=O	1850 ~ 1650	strong
C—O	1275 ~ 1050	strong
C—N	1400 ~ 1020	medium
O—H (alcohol)	3650 ~ 3200	strong, broad
O—H (carboxylic acid)	3300 ~ 2500	strong, very broad
N—H	3500 ~ 3100	medium, broad
C—H	3300 ~ 2700	medium

Infared Spectroscopy testing equipment and testing methods commonly used.

5. 2. 1 Fourier transform infrared spectrometers

Almost all modern IR spectrometers use the Fourier transform method to scan the full spectral range at the same time. This method has some obvious advantages. A further advantage is that it is possible to get a spectrum from very small or very dilute samples by performing multiple scans and adding the data to improve the signal-to-noise ratio.

5. 2. 2 Sample

There are a variety of techniques for sample preparation dependent on the physical form of the sample to be analyzed.

5. 2. 2. 1 Solids

There are two methods for sample preparation involving the use of Nujol mull or potassium bromide disks.

5. 2. 2. 2 Liquids

Liquid samples can be sandwiched between two plates of a high purity salt (commonly sodium chloride, or common salt, although a number of other salts such as potassium bromide or calcium fluoride are also used) . The plates are transparent to the infrared light.

5. 2. 2. 3 Gases

To obtain an infrared spectrum of a gas requires the use of a cylindrical gas cell with windows at each end composed of an infrared inactive material such as KBr, NaCl, or CaF_2. The cell usually has an inlet and outlet port with a tap to enable the cell to be easily filled with the gas to be analyzed.

5.2.3 Mass spectrometry （MS）

Mass spectrometry is an analytical tool used for measuring the molecular mass of a sample. It uses a very small amount of sample and provides the molecular weight and valuable information about the molecular formula, High-resolution mass spectrometry （HRMS） can provide an accurate molecular formula.

All mass spectrometers require the sample compound to be ionized and those ions to be transferred into the gas phase for analysis: this may be a simultaneous process or a distinct series of events. A mass spectrometer ionizes molecules in a high vacuum, sorts the ion according to their masses, and records the abundance of ion of each mass. A mass spectrum is then plotted.

The ion sources commonly used in MS include electron ionization （EI）, chemical ionization （CI）, fast-atom bombardment （FAB）, etc. We will discuss some the most common techniques.

5.2.3.1 Electron ionization （EI）

The analyte of interest is vaporized and solids are introduced on a hot probe, liquids via a heated septum and bleed valve, and gases through a membrane or a needle valve system. The vapour is crossed by an electron beam, which have high-energy electrons （usually 70eV）. Analyte molecules absorb some of this energy （typically around 20eV） and this causes a number of processes to occur. The simplest of these is where the analyte is ionized by the removal of single electron. This yields a radical cation, termed the molecular ion （$M^+ \cdot$）, the m/z of which corresponds to the molecular weight of the analyte. This method is the most often used, but the weak or absent M^+ peak which could inhibit determination of molecular weight, and the other disadvantage is that the molecules must be vaporized and thermally stable during vaporization.

5.2.3.2 Chemical impact ionization （CI）

Ionization begins when a reagent gas （R） is ionized by electron impact and then subsequently reacts with analyte molecules （M） to produce analyte ions. This method gives molecular weight information and reduced fragmentation in comparison to EI.

5.2.3.3 Fast atom bombardment （FAB）

This method requires samples to be dissolved in a matrix such as glycerol and therefore the sample must be inserted on a probe system. The surface of this mixture is subjected to a beam of energetic xenon ［or argon］ atoms which sputter ions from the mixture. These may be positive or negative and each can be detected separately.

5.2.3.4 Matrix assisted laser desorption ionization （MALDI）

This method works on solid sample spots co-deposited with a light-absorbing matrix. By irradiating these sample spots in the matrix with high intensity laster radiation, both positive and negative ions, are produced.

5.2.3.5 High-resolution mass spectrometry （HRMS）

HRMS can be used to determine a molecular formula. It can use extra stages of electrostatic or magnetic focusing to form a very precise beam and to detect particle masses to an accuracy of about 1/2000. A mass determined to several significant figures using an HRMS is called an exact mass, which can identify the correct formula of the molecular.

5.2.4 Nuclear magnetic resonance spectroscopy （NMR）

Over the past five decades nuclear magnetic resonance spectroscopy （NMR）, has become the very effective techniques for determining the structure of organic compounds. NMR like the IR, needs a little sample, it is also non-destructive. Many structures you can estimate by the NMR alone, while many complex compounds, you must use some other methods. (Fig 1-10 see the Chinse part.)

In principle, NMR is applicable to any nucleus possessing spin. The nuclei of many elemental isotopes have a characteristic spin (I). Some nuclei have integral spins (e. g. $I = 1, 2, 3\cdots$), some have fractional spins (e. g. $I = 1/2, 3/2, 5/2\cdots$), and a few have no spin, $I = 0$. The most important nuclei in organic chemistry are ^1H, ^{13}C, ^{19}F and ^{31}P, all of which have $I = 1/2$. The most important applications for the organic chemist are proton ^1H-NMR and ^{13}C-NMR spectroscopy.

As we all know a nucleus of spin I will have $2I + 1$ possible orientation. So in existence of an external magnetic field, nucleus with spin 1/2 will have two spin states, $+1/2$ and $-1/2$. The difference in energy is always very small between the two spin states and dependent on the external magnetic field strength. The two spin states have the same energy when the external field is zero, but in non-zero magnetic field they have different energies. (Fig 1-11 see the Chinse part.)

^1H-NMR provides following information.

5. 2. 4. 1 Chemical shift (δ)

Chemists compare the chemical shifts of the hydrogen atoms in an organic molecule with it of the hydrogen in the standard substance that can be used to compare the shielding of hydrogen in the molecule. The standard substance is tetramethylsilane, $(CH_3)_4Si$, which is abbreviated as TMS. δ (ppm) often stands for chemical shifts. For example, in the ^1H-NMR of ethanol (CH_3CH_2OH), three characteristic sets of signals corresponds to three typical chemical shifts, which are a methyl signal, a methylene signal and a hydroxyl signal, respectively. The chemical shift of the methyl characteristic peak is 1 ppm, the chemical shift of the methylene group attached to the hydroxyl group is about 4 ppm, and the hydroxyl group is between 2 and 3 ppm depending on the solvent used. The shape and size of the peak are also indexes for identifying the structure of the compound. As shown in the above example of the spectrum for ethanol, the peak area of methyl is three times than it of hydroxyl. Similarly, the peak area of methylene twice bigger than hydroxyl, but only 2/3 of methyl. Chemical shifts of common protons are showed in Fig. 1-12 (see the Chinse part.)

5. 2. 4. 2 Spin-spin Coupling

We know that nuclei are equivalent in the same chemical environment or with the same chemical shift, while they are not equivalent in different chemical environments or with different chemical shifts. Closed adjacent nuclei have the effect on effective magnetic fields of each other that leads to appearance of many group peaks produced by the chemically unequal nucleus in the NMR spectrum. This kind of effect is called spin-spin coupling, which provides the detailed information to analyze the connection among atoms in a molecule. General law for the proton splitting in the NMR spectrum used to judge is shown as following: the amount of splitting peaks is $n + 1$, n represents the number of adjacent equivalent protons: no ortho proton, a singlet (s); one adjacent proton is doublet (d); two adjacent protons are triplet (t); three adjacent protons are quadruple (q). For example, in the proton NMR of ethanol mentioned above, methyl protons are coupled by the ortho methylene protons and split into triplet peaks with an intensity ratio of 1 : 2 : 1; similarly, methylene protons are ortho coupled by methyl protons and split into fourfold peaks with an intensity ratio of 1 : 3 : 3 : 1.

IV. The Design Ideas and Implementation Methods of Designing Experimengs

（E. g. The extraction, isolation and identification of psoralen and isopsoralene）

1. Origination of medicinal herbs

Malaytea Scurfpea Fruit, the seeds of *Psoralea corylifolia* L. It has the effects of warming kidney to invigorate yang, antidiarrhea and used as drug of impotence and seminal emission, enuresis, frequent micturition, knee-waist pain, and deficiency of the kidney. The main chemical constituents of Malaytea Scurfpea Fruit are psoralen, isopsoralen and flavonoids.

2. Experiment purpose

2.1 To learn the main access to the major domestic and foreign literature of natural product chemistry.

2.2 To learn the methods of collecting literature and writing review.

2.3 After analyzing the literature and combining with the existing knowledge, the methods of extraction, separation and identification of psoralen and isopsoralen were designed and fulfilled.

2.4 To learn and master the methods of isolation and structural identification of the coumarins.

3. Experiment arrangements

3.1 Access to literature and write a review

Foreign literature: Scifinder Scholar, CA CD-ROM databases, Medline and other databases.

Chinese literature: CD-ROM database retrieval Chinese medicine, Chinese biomedical databases and so on.

The purpose is learning to consult systematically domestic and foreign literature with detailed records and write a review, the main contents are as following.

3. 1. 1 The plant origin, species, genus and distribution of Malaytea Scurfpea Fruit.

3. 1. 2 Clinical and pharmacological activity of Malaytea Scurfpea Fruit, psoralen and isopsoralen.

3. 1. 3 The name, melting point, structure, physical and chemical properties, extraction, isolation and structural identification of the main compounds in Malaytea Scurfpea Fruit.

3. 2 Communication literature and design experimental programs

Request to exchange and discuss the literature sufficiently, and then design the experiment proposal with group as the unit program, the main contents are as following.

3. 2. 1 The methods, devices and solvents of the extraction.

3. 2. 2 The methods, devices and solvents of the purification.

3. 2. 3 The methods of the separation, the type, amount of the chromatography and the species, ratio, and amount of the eluant.

3. 2. 4 List the required experimental materials and arrange the schedule.

3. 3 Implement of the experimental proposal

Under the guidance of teachers, fulfill the experiment independently according to the established experimental proposal. Require to obtain the monomer compounds of psoralen and isopsoralen respectively (no less than 5mg) after the extraction and purification within a specified period of time (such as three weeks). If there any adjustments, please notify the instructor promptly so that the necessary experimental materials could be provided in order to ensure the experiment smoothly proceeds. Then the physico-chemical properties and necessary spectrum of the isolated monomer compounds should be determined.

3.4 Discussion of the experimental

Firstly, the experimental records should be finished each group, then the experimental results be discussed and the gain and loss be summarized. Secondly, further discussion focus on the whole class and the quality of the products be checked, experience of experimental operation be exchanged, and fit and unfit of different experimental plans be compared.

3.5 Complete the test reports

The whole experimental process should be discussed, the success and failure of the experiment be introduced, merits and demerits of different experimental plans be evaluated, and improvements be proposed. The test report will be completed eventually.

第二部分　天然药物化学实验实例

实验一　基础实验

一、天然化合物的重结晶和样品的干燥

扫码"学一学"

1. **简介**　天然化合物经分离纯化后，最后一步是将目标化合物制备成有用的形式，即制备纯化合物的饱和溶液，使析出结晶，处理得干燥固体。结晶和重结晶可视为纯化的过程，也常用来制备单晶，经 X - 射线单晶衍射法来确定分子的结构。

样品在干燥状态下较稳定，另外，收率的计算及化合物结构的确定均需使样品处于干燥状态。

2. **目的**
（1）掌握重结晶的基本操作方法。
（2）熟悉天然化合物的常用干燥方法。

3. **操作方法**　称取酒石酸（DL - 酒石酸，m. p. 204℃）0.01g，置于 25ml 圆底烧瓶中加入 10 ml 水或乙醇使其溶解（必要时可将混合物加热以溶解）。若有固体物质残留，可用菊形滤纸过滤，滤液静置，冷至室温，结晶析出。抽滤，收集产物。将固体放在表面皿上干燥，称重。测熔点。计算收率。

记录：_____ 克，熔点_____，收率_____。

二、TLC 铺板、干燥和活化

扫码"看一看"

1. **简介**　薄层色谱中的吸附剂是铺在玻璃、塑料、金属片或薄板上的较薄的、均匀的一层细粉状物质，因支持剂的种类、制备方法和选用溶剂的不同，可按吸附、分配或二者结合的方式达到分离化合物的目的。可以通过比较斑点的 R_f 值，或将未知样品与对照品在同一板上展开至同样高度，对样品进行初步的鉴定。还可通过比较可见斑点的大小进行半定量的判断或可以通过光密度测量法实现定量测定。

TLC 中涂布的物质与柱色谱用的吸附剂非常相似，如硅胶、氧化铝、聚酰胺等，只是它们的颗粒更细一些，一般直径为 5 ~ 40μm。有些还含有石膏、淀粉等黏合剂以增强涂层与薄板的黏合力。有时里面还含有荧光指示剂（如硅酸锌等），在 254nm 或 365 nm 的紫外光下能显示荧光，可借此对分离的斑点进行检测。到目前为止，硅胶是最常用的薄层色谱吸附剂。

在涂布吸附剂时，用于排列和放置薄板的排列盘和具有平整表面的薄板是必需的。而涂布器也很常用，当它从玻璃板上移过时，会在板的表面均匀铺上所需厚度的吸附剂涂层。

2. **目的**　掌握硅胶薄层色谱板的制备方法。

3. **仪器和试剂** 玻璃板（5 cm×10 cm 或 2.5 cm×7.5 cm，洁净且干燥）、薄层色谱用硅胶 H、0.8% 羧甲基纤维素钠（CMC－Na）水溶液

4. **实验步骤**

（1）把玻璃板在排列盘中依次相邻放好，置涂布器于其中一端。

（2）在三角烧瓶中把一份硅胶 H 和三份 CMC－Na 溶液混合，并用玻棒搅匀直至没有气泡。

（3）把混好的糊倒入涂布器中，并均匀地移动涂布器至排列盘的另一端后，移开涂布器。

（4）铺好的板静置 5 分钟，然后把它们面朝上移至一个水平平面上，阴干。

（5）把阴干后的板置于 105℃的烘箱中烘 30 分钟。

（6）待板凉至室温后，置干燥器中保存。

三、色谱用硅胶柱的填装以及硅胶柱色谱法分离四季青中酚酸类成分实例

（一）色谱用硅胶柱的填装

1. **简介** 液相柱色谱可以是液－固色谱或液－液色谱。如果固定相是吸附剂，也称为液相吸附色谱；若为离子交换物质，就称为离子交换色谱；若为非离子的聚合物，如聚苯乙烯或 Sephadex，则称为凝胶渗透色谱、凝胶过滤色谱或分子排阻色谱。在柱中或纸上的液－液分配色谱可以进一步分为正相分配色谱（极性固定液）和反相分配色谱（固定相非极性）。

对于液相吸附色谱来说，固定相是填入柱中的表面活性固体（如氧化铝、硅胶和活性炭等），流动相由一种或几种有机溶剂混合组成。混合物中的不同组分由于与固定相吸附力的不同而得以分离。被弱吸附的物质移动得快而被强吸附的物质移动受到阻滞。与吸附力有关的分子间作用因表面吸附剂、被吸附物质和溶剂的性质（极性）不同可有多种形式。硅胶和氧化铝是目前为止最常用的液相吸附色谱的吸附剂。

吸附剂的吸附能力用活度来衡量。活度可分为五级（表 2－1），广泛认为其与吸附剂、被吸附物质和能产生这种吸附的位置的个数有关。一级活度是最高的，对硅胶来说可以在不超过 300℃的温度下加热数小时达到。向其中加入适量的水可以进一步降低其活度到 Ⅱ～Ⅴ。可以用特定染料的色谱行为来判断吸附剂的活度等级。

表 2－1 硅胶的活度与含水量之间的关系

硅胶的含水量（重量百分比）	0	5	15	25	38
活度（依次降低）	I	II	III	IV	V

吸附柱色谱中常用的填充方法有湿法装柱和干法装柱。

2. **目的**

（1）了解测定硅胶的活度及硅胶减活的方法。

（2）掌握硅胶色谱柱的填充方法。

3. **仪器和试剂** 色谱用玻璃柱、3 mm×105 mm 玻璃管、层析用硅胶、0.02%～0.05% 对二甲氨基偶氮苯，苯。

4. 实验步骤

1）硅胶活度的测定

①取一个 3 mm × 105 mm 玻璃管，用棉花封住一端，从另一端向内加入待测活度的硅胶，同时轻敲玻璃管，使管内充满吸附剂。

②配制 0.02% ~ 0.05% 的对二氨甲基偶氮苯的苯溶液。

③将上述溶液滴于棉花上，置玻璃管于一小试管中，用苯展开。

④当溶剂到达管的顶端时取出玻璃管，观察色带位置并计算染料的 R_f 值。

⑤根据表 2 - 2 计算硅胶的活度。

表 2 - 2　硅胶活度的测定

染料的比移值	0.15	0.55	0.65
硅胶的含水量（重量百分比）	0	12	15
活度	Ⅰ	Ⅱ	Ⅲ

2）硅胶的减活

①用上法测定所用硅胶的活度。

②根据硅胶的质量和要达到的活度计算减活所需加入水的体积。

③把水加入到盛有硅胶的三角烧瓶中，密封，不断用力振摇。

④1 小时后测定减活后的硅胶的活度。

3）色谱用硅胶柱的填装

①将一小团玻璃丝或脱脂棉放于柱底部使形成一个较松的垫层。

②一边轻敲柱子的外侧，一边将硅胶慢慢倒入柱子中。

③打开活塞，让一种非极性的烃类溶剂流过柱体，直至整个柱床全部润湿。关闭活塞备用。

（二）硅胶柱色谱法分离四季青中酚酸类成分实例

1. 实验原理　四季青 *Ilex purpurea* Hassk. 是冬青科冬青属植物，分布于我国长江以南各地，其根、叶均可制药，主要功效是清热解毒、生肌敛疮、活血止血。

原儿茶醛（protocatechuic aldehyde；3，4 - 二羟基苯甲醛）是四季青叶中抗心绞痛的主要有效成分之一，具有扩张冠状动脉，增加冠脉血流量的作用。该化合物熔点 153 ~ 154 ℃，易溶于乙醇、丙酮、醋酸乙酯、乙醚和热水，溶于冷水，不溶于苯和三氯甲烷。有引湿性，在水中易氧化变色。

原儿茶酸（protocatechuic acid；3，4 - 二羟基苯甲酸）存在于冬青科植物冬青的叶等植物中。白色至褐色结晶性粉末，在空气中变色。熔点 198 ~ 200 ℃，易溶于水、乙醇、乙醚、丙酮和乙酸乙酯，难溶于苯和三氯甲烷。具有抗菌作用，体外试验时对绿脓杆菌、大肠埃希菌、伤寒杆菌、痢疾杆菌、产碱杆菌及枯草杆菌和金黄色葡萄球菌均有不同程度的抑菌作用。亦有祛痰、平喘作用。临床用于治疗慢性气管炎。

2，4 - 二硝基苯肼（2，4 - dinitrophenylhydrazine）红色结晶性粉末，熔点 197 ~ 198 ℃，微溶于水、乙醇，溶于酸。用于炸药制造，可用作化学试剂用于鉴别醛、酮。与其生成的 2，4 - 二硝基苯腙为黄色或红色晶体易于观察。

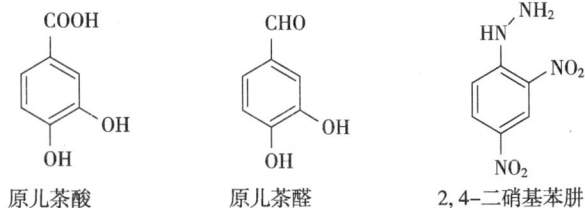

原儿茶酸　　　　　　原儿茶醛　　　　　2,4-二硝基苯肼

2. 实验目的

（1）初步了解天然产物的分离，检出，鉴定方法。

（2）熟悉柱层析的基本操作。

3. 操作步骤

（1）装柱　硅胶（100～200目，活度：Ⅴ级）6 g，干法装柱。

（2）上样　样品用移液管吸取1ml加入柱顶。

（3）洗脱　石油醚/乙酸乙酯（4∶6），约30 ml，小漏斗加入。

（4）收集　用小三角瓶按色带收集，经验为每6 ml收集一次，结果较为理想。

（5）检出　取硅胶CMC-Na小板，在板上如图画小格，用毛细管吸取各分洗脱液分别滴在各小格内，然后用毛细管取检出试剂滴在检品处，上行做空白对照，下行做反应。当检出洗脱液至无腙的橙色斑点出现时改用氨性硝酸银试剂检出原儿茶酸。当正反应时应使银-氨络离子的溶液中的银离子被原儿茶酸的邻二酚烃基还原成金属银呈黑色斑点反应。

（6）TLC检出　将上述流份分别点样进行薄层层析检出。薄层层析条件如下。

①硅胶板　硅胶CMC-Na薄层板

②展开剂　三氯甲烷∶丙酮∶甲醇∶乙酸=7∶2∶0.5∶0.5

③显色剂　2%的三氯化铁乙醇溶液显色。

（7）合并流份　按薄层层析结果合并相同流份。

（8）判断　将层析柱洗净放入烘箱内。记录各流份的原位显色反应及薄层层析的结果（绘出图谱），以初步判断各流分中所含成分。

四、讨论

1. 为何在铺板之前，色谱用的玻璃板要完全洗净并干燥？

2. 为何铺好的TLC板用前要在烘箱中干燥？

3. 实验室的工作人员总是尽量避免使流动相液面低于色谱柱中吸附剂的上端，为什么？

扫码"练一练"

Part Ⅱ   Examples for Natural Pharmaceutical Chemistry Experiments

Experiment Ⅰ   Basic Experiment

Ⅰ. Recrystallization of Natural Compounds and Drying of Samples

1. Introduction

The hard work has been done and the purification is "complete" -the target compound has been separated. The final step is to prepare the target compound in a usable form. This generally means producing a concentrated solution of pure compound or the pure dry solid. The process of crystallization or recrystallization can be used as a purification step or used to produce crystals for molecular structure determination by single-crystal X-ray diffraction.

The compound is more likely to remain stable in a dry form. In order to determine the yield of isolated, it usually needs to be weighed as a dry solid. In many cases, the aim of the purification will be to carry out spectroscopy in order to elucidate molecular structure.

2. Purpose

From this experiment, students will master the basic procedures of recrystallization and be familiar with the drying methods of natural compounds.

3. Procedure

Weigh out 0. 01g tartaric acid, transfer it to a 25 ml round-bottomed flask and add 10ml water or ethanol . Warm the mixture to make it dissolve as it is necessary. If there is solid undissolved, filter with a fluted filter paper, filtrate is cooled to room temperature undisturbed when the product has separated completely, collect the crystals with suction on a Hirsch funnel. Spread the crystals on a watch glass, allow them to dry thoroughly, weigh the amounts of crystals and calculate the percentage recovery and determine the melting point of the purified products.

Record: _____ g, m. p. _____ , Yield: _____ .

Ⅱ. Preparation, Drying and Activation of Silica TLC

In TLC (thin-layer chromatography), the adsorbent is a relatively thin, uniform layer of finely powdered material applied to a glass, plastic, or mental sheet or plate, glass plates being commonly employed. The separations achieved may be based upon adsorption, partition, or a combination of both effects, depending on the particular type of support, its preparation, and its use with different solvents. Presumptive identification can be effected by observation of spot of identical R_f value and about equal magnitude obtained, respectively, with an unknown and a references sample chromatographed on the same plate. A visual comparison of the size of the spots may serve for semiquantitative analysis. Quantitative measurements are possible by means of densitometry.

The coating materials of TLC are similar to the sorbents used for column chromatography except that they are generally of a smaller particle size, such as silica, alumina, polyamide etc., normally 5 to 40 μm in diameter. Some of those contain a binder such as plaster of Paris (CaSO₄) or starch to improve the adherence of the film to the plate. An inert fluorescent indicator (e. g. zinc silicate) which fluoresces when illuminated with 254 or 365 nm UV light so as to aid in the detection of separated spots is also sometimes including. Silica is by far the most used adsorbent for TLC.

An aligning tray and a flat surface upon must be employed which to align and rest the plates during the application of the adsorbent. A spreader is also always used also, which will apply a uniform layer of adsorbent of desired thickness over the entire surface of the plate, when move over the glass plate.

2. Purpose

Acquire the preparation of silica thin-layer chromatography.

3. Apparatus and reagents

(1) Glass plates (5 cm × 10 cm or 2.5 cm × 7.5 cm, clean and dry)

(2) Silica H for TLC.

(3) 0.75% CMC-Na.

4. Procedures

(1) Arrange the plates on the aligning tray adjacent each other. Position the spreader on the end of plate.

(2) Mix 1 part of silica H with 3 part of CMC-Na solution uniformly by shaking vigorously for 30 seconds in a glass-stoppered conical flask.

(3) Transfer the slurry to the spreader. Draw the spreader smoothly over the plates toward another end of the aligning tray, and remove the spreader when it reaches the end.

(4) Allow the plates to remain undisturbed for 5 minutes, and then transfer the square, layers up, to an even plane until dry in the shade.

(5) Transfer the dried plates to drying oven, and activate at 105 ℃ for 30 minutes.

(6) Allow them to cool to room temperature, and store the plates in a desiccator.

III. Preparation of Silica Column for Chromatography and the Isolation of Phenols from *Ilex chinensis* Sims by silica gel CC

I) Preparation of Silica Column for Chromatography

1. Introduction of liquid column chromatography

Liquid chromatography in columns can be liquid-solid chromatography (LSC) or liquid-liquid (partition) chromatography (LLC). If the solid stationary phase is an adsorbent, the process is called liquid adsorption chromatography. If it is an ion-exchange material, it is termed ion-exchange chromatography (IXC). If it is nonionic polymer, e. g. polystyrene or Sephadex, the term gel permeation chromatography, gel filtration chromatography or molecular exclusion chromatography is used. Liquid-liquid (partition) chromatography (LLC) in column or on paper may be further subdivided into normal-phase partition chromatography (fixed polar liquids) and reversed-phase partition chromatography（fixed nor-polar liquids）.

For liquid column adsorption chromatography, the stationary phase is a surface-active solid（e. g., alumina, silica or charcoal）packed into a column, and the mobile phase is a solvent composed of one or more organic liquids. The separation of a mixture results from the different adsorption of components onto the surface of the solid. Weakly adsorbed solutes travel more quickly while strongly adsorbed solutes are retarded. The molecular interactions involved in adsorption can be of several types depending upon the nature（polarity）of the surface, the adsorbed solutes, and the solvent. Silica and alumina is by far the most commonly used adsorbent for liquid adsorption chromatography.

The adsorptive capability of adsorbent is evaluated by its activity, which is classified into five grades（Table 2 −1）, and is broadly regarded as relating both to the adsorbent and the molecules being adsorbed, and to the number of sites at which such attraction takes places. Grade I is the most active, and is obtained by heating for several hours at temperatures not exceeding 300℃ for silica. Successively less active grade, II ~ V, are obtained by the addition of appropriate amounts of water. The activity grade is assessed by determining the chromatogramphic behavior of specified dyes.

Table 2 −1   The relationship between activity grade with the percent of water in silica gel

Percent（by weight）of Water Added to Silica	0	5	15	25	38
Resulting Grades（decreasing activity）	I	II	III	IV	V

The generally methods of packing most adsorptions in a column are slurry, or dry packing.

2. Purposes

2. 1 Learn how to determine and degrade the activity of silica.

2. 2 Acquire the preparation of silica column for chromatography.

3. Apparatus and reagent

Glass tube for chromatography, 3 mm × 105 mm Glass tube, Silica for chromatography, 0. 02% ~0. 05% p-Dimethylamino-azobenzene, Benzene

4. Procedures

4. 1 The determination of activity for silica.

4. 1. 1 Hinder one end of a 3 mm × 105 mm glass tube with a roll of cotton. Add silica used from another end while beating the tube to make it is full of the adsorbent.

4. 1. 2 Prepare the solution of benzene containing p-dimethylamino-azobenzene 0. 02% ~ 0. 05%.

4. 1. 3 Drop the solution on the cotton and put the tube in a corvette, then develop the tube by benzene.

4. 1. 4 Take out the tube when the solvent reaches the top of tube, observe the position and calculate the R_f value of the dyes.

4. 1. 5 Estimate the activity of the silica according to Table 2 −2.

Table 2 – 2　The Determination of Activity for Silica

The R_f value of the dyes	0. 15	0. 55	0. 65
Percent（by weight）of Water in Silica	0	12	15
Resulting Grades	I	II	III

4. 2 The Deactivating of Silica

4. 2. 1 Determine the activity grade of the silica used according to the method mentioned above.

4. 2. 2 Calculate the volume of water need adding to degrade the activity of silica basesd on the weight of silica and the activity to be reaching.

4. 2. 3 Add the water to silica on a conical flask, seal, shake vigorously at times.

4. 2. 4 Determine the grade of the deactivated silica after 1 hour.

4. 3 The Preparation of Silica Column for Chromatography by Dry-packing.

4. 3. 1 Force a small piece of glass wool or pledged down the column so as to form a loose pad at the bottom.

4. 3. 2 Slowly fill the column with silica while the sides of the column are gently tapped.

4. 3. 3 A nonpolar, hydrocarbon solvent is passed down the column with the stopcock open until the entire column is wet. Close the plunger, wait for using.

Ⅱ）The Isolation of Phenols from *Ilex chinensis* Sims by silica gel CC

1. Principle

Ilex purpurea Hassk. , the plant from genus *Ilex*, is distributed around the south of the Yangtze River in China. Its root and leaves can be used as traditional Chinesse medicine. It has the role of clearing heat and renuiing toxin, producing the muscle and healing ulcer, promoting blood circulation and arresting bleeding.

Protocatechuic aldehyde（3,4-dihydroxybenzaldehyde）is one of the main effective constituents to cure angina from the leaves of *Ilex chinensis* Sims. It shows the activity to expand coronary artery, and increase coronary blood flow. Protocatechuic aldehyde, m. p. 153 ~ 154 ℃, dissolves in ethyl alcohol, acetone, ethyl acetate, diethyl ether and hot water, also able to dissolves in cold water, slightly soluble in benzene and chloroform. It has the hygroscopicity, and change color in water, oxidized.

Existed in leaves of*Ilex chinensis* Sims of *Ilex* family, protocatechuic acid（3,4-dihydroxybenzoic acid）is white to brownish crystalline powder, change color in air. , m. p. 198 ~ 200℃. Protocatechuic acid dissolves in water, alcohol, diethyl ether, acetone, ethyl acetate easily. It's slightly soluble in benzene and chloroform. In vitro tests, protocatechuic acid shows the antibacterial action to various microorganisms, such as *Pseudomonas aeruginosa*, *Escherichia coli*, *Typhoid bacillus*, *Dysentery bacillus*, *Alcaligenes faecalis*, *Bacillus subtilis* and *Staphylococcus aureus*. It also shows the expectorant effect and anti-asthma activity.

2, 4-dinitrophenylhydrazine, red crystalline powder, m. p. 197 ~ 198 ℃, slightly soluble in water and ethanol, dissolves in acid, can be used to make explosive. It can be used to identify aldehydes and ketones, producing 2, 4-dinitrobenzene hydrazine, yellow or red crystal, easily to be observed.

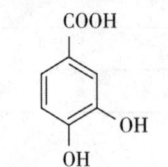

protocatechuic acid   Protocatechuic aldehyde   2,4−dinitrophenylhydrazine

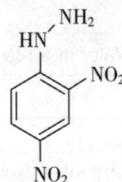

2. Purpose

2. 1 Preliminarily know the isolation, detection and identification methods of natural compounds.

2. 2 Be familiar with the basic operation of column chromatography (CC).

3. Procedures

3. 1 Filling column: fill little cotton in the bottom of column, add dry silica (6g, Grade V) into column.

3. 2 Loading sample: add 1ml solution of extracts into column using transfer pipette.

3. 3 Eluting: add eluents (PE-EtOAc, 4 : 6) 30ml by little funnel.

3. 4 Collecting: collect eluents according to detection of spot reaction. Empirically, the eluate is collected every 6 ml, and the result is ideal.

3. 5 Detection: Draw little grids in thin layer plate as picture shows, each eluent was dripped in grids applying with microcapillary, detection regents was dripped at the same place, up as blank control, down as reaction point. As orange spot appears, change the detection regent to be ammoniacal silver nitrate reagent to detect protocatechuic acid. When the action is positive, silver ammonia complex ion will be reduced to be silver, as black spot appears, by adjacent two phenolic hydroxyl of protocatechuic acid.

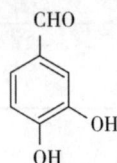

3. 6 TLC examine: The fractions above-mentioned were applied with microcapilllary, developed by the condition as follows:

Silica gel CMC-Na thin layer plate

Developing solvent: ($CHCl_3$: acetone : CH_3OH : CH_3COOH, 7 : 2 : 0. 5 : 0. 5)

Chromagenic reagent: $FeCl_3$/EtOH solutions

3. 7 Combine the same fractions according to the result of thin layer chromatography.

3. 8 Clean the column and put in drying oven. Recording the drop reaction of each fraction and result of thin layer chromatography (draw down the plate), preliminarily judge what compounds are in each fraction.

IV. Questions

1. Why should the glass plate for TLC be thoroughly washed and dry before coating it?

2. Why are the TLC plates oven dried before use?

3. Why are laboratory workers are usually cautioned not to allow the liquid level to drop below the top of a column of adsorbent?

实验二 芦丁和槲皮素的提取、分离和结构鉴定

扫码"学一学"

一、简介

芦丁也称芸香苷，广泛存在于植物界，在槐花米和荞麦叶中含量较高。槐花米系豆科植物槐 *Sophora japonica* L. 的花蕾，古时用作止血药，常用作提取芦丁的原料。

芦丁有减少毛细血管通透性的作用，临床上主要用于高血压的辅助治疗，对于放射线伤害引起的出血症也有一定的作用。

槲皮素是芦丁的苷元，广泛存在于水果（如柑橘）和许多食物如荞麦、洋葱等植物中，具有显著地抗炎作用。槲皮素可由芦丁水解制得。

二、目的

1. 掌握黄酮类成分的提取分离方法。
2. 熟悉黄酮类成分的主要化学性质。
3. 掌握用薄层色谱或纸色谱鉴定黄酮苷及其苷元和糖的方法。

三、原理

芦丁为淡黄色、细小针状结晶，含 3 个结晶水，熔点 177～178℃。芦丁可溶于热水（1∶200），难溶于冷水（1∶8000），易溶于热甲醇（1∶7）、冷甲醇（1∶100）、热乙醇（1∶30）和冷乙醇（1∶300），难溶于乙酸乙酯、丙酮，不溶于苯、三氯甲烷、乙醚及石油醚等非极性有机溶剂。芦丁结构中有多个酚羟基，显弱酸性，故易溶于碱液并呈黄色，酸化后又析出。因此，可用"碱提酸沉"法进行提取。

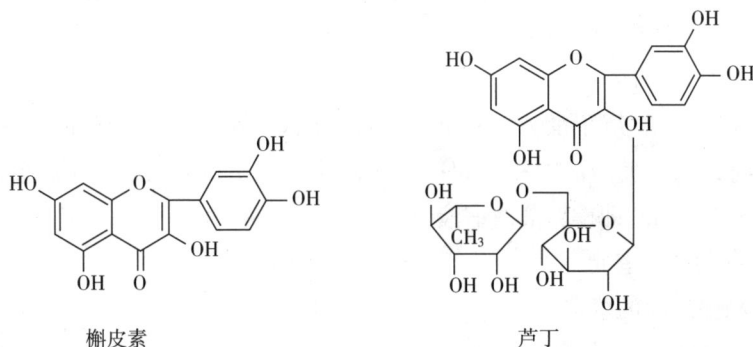

槲皮素　　　　　　　　　　　　芦丁

槲皮素亦为黄色结晶，熔点 313～314℃。槲皮素溶于热乙醇（1∶23），冷乙醇（1∶300），还可溶于冰醋酸、乙酸乙酯、丙酮等溶剂，但不溶于石油醚、苯、乙醚、三氯甲烷和水。

四、仪器与试剂

1. **仪器**　烧杯（100ml，500ml），圆底烧瓶（100ml，150ml），抽滤瓶（500ml），冷凝管，循环水泵，紫外灯，展开缸，点样毛细管（1mm），布氏漏斗，长颈漏斗。

2. **试剂**　0.4% 硼砂水，石灰乳，2% 硫酸，盐酸，氢氧化钡，三氯化铝，乙醇，甲醇，聚酰胺薄膜，滤纸。

五、展开剂及对照品

1. **展开剂** 正丁醇∶醋酸∶水（4∶1∶5 或 4∶1∶1，上层），25% 醋酸，85% 醋酸，乙醇∶水（7∶3），氨水。

2. **对照品** 芦丁，槲皮素，葡萄糖，鼠李糖。

六、操作方法

1. 芦丁的提取和纯化

（1）提取 槐花米 20g，置于 500ml 烧杯中，加 0.4% 硼砂水的沸腾溶液 250ml，此时溶液 pH 约为 8。不断搅拌，并不断以石灰乳调节并始终保持提取液 pH 为 8，加热，保持微沸 30min，另外，加热提取过程中以蒸馏水补充失去的水。静置 5~10min，使其凉至室温，倾出上清液，过滤。药渣以同样方法重复提取一次。合并滤液，用盐酸将滤液调至 pH 2~3 左右，滴加 8 滴乙酸乙酯，放置过夜使析出沉淀。抽滤，水洗沉淀 3~4 次，放置空气中自然干燥得芦丁粗品。称重，计算得率。

扫码"看一看"

（2）芦丁的重结晶 取芦丁粗品 1g，用 200ml 水加热溶解，此过程中不必补水，当芦丁全部溶解后，趁热抽滤，放置滤液使析出结晶，抽滤，滤出结晶。母液浓缩至一半体积，放置又析出结晶，抽滤后，合并两次结晶，用乙醇重结晶一次，得精制芦丁。干燥称重，计算得率。

2. 芦丁的酸水解

称取芦丁 0.6 g，置于 100ml 圆底烧瓶中，加 2% H_2SO_4 40ml，小火加热，微沸回流 1h。溶液逐渐由澄清变浑浊，析出细小的黄色针状结晶。反应结束后，放冷，抽滤（注意：保留滤液 20 ml，以检查其中所含单糖）。抽滤，得到结晶，即槲皮素粗品。

扫码"看一看"

将槲皮素粗品置于 100ml 圆底烧瓶中，加 50% 乙醇 50ml，加热回流使溶解，趁热抽滤，滤液转移至三角烧瓶中，放置析晶，抽滤，得精制槲皮素。减压下于 110℃ 干燥可得无水槲皮素，熔点 313~314℃。

3. 糖液的处理

取芦丁酸水解时时保留的滤液 20ml，置于 50 ml 烧杯中，分次加 Ba(OH)$_2$ 细粉约 2.6g，使溶液中和至 pH 7，滤除生成的 BaSO$_4$ 沉淀，使用菊形滤纸常压过滤，滤液浓缩至 1~2 ml 即得糖液浓缩液。

4. 黄酮及糖的薄层鉴定

（1）芦丁和槲皮素的鉴定

1）方法一 硅胶薄层色谱

①滤纸 新华一号层析用滤纸（5cm×8cm）。

②样品溶液 自制芦丁及槲皮素少量，以适量乙醇加热（或超声）溶解。

③对照品溶液 芦丁及槲皮素标准品适量，以适量乙醇加热（或超声）溶解。

④展开剂 正丁醇–醋酸–水（4∶1∶5 上层或 4∶1∶1）。

用毛细管各吸取样品和对照溶液适量，点于 TLC 薄层板上，用上述展开剂展开。吹干溶剂后，在可见光及紫外灯（365nm）下观察色斑，用 AlCl$_3$ 或浓氨水熏后再在可见光及紫外灯（365nm）下分别观察色斑变化。

2）方法二 聚酰胺薄层色谱法

①样品溶液 自制及标准品芦丁及槲皮素少量，以适量乙醇溶解。

②展开剂　乙醇 – 水（7∶3）。

用毛细管各吸取样品和对照品溶液适量，点于聚酰胺薄层上，用上述展开剂展开。展开剂吹干后，在可见光及紫外光下观察色斑，用 AlCl₃ 或浓氨水熏滤纸后再在可见光及紫外光下分别观察色斑变化。

（2）糖的纸色谱鉴定

①滤纸　色谱用滤纸（5cm×8cm）。

②样品溶液的制备　取芦丁酸水解时保留的滤液 20 ml，置于 50 ml 烧杯中，分次加 Ba(OH)₂ 细粉约 2.6 g，使溶液中和至 pH 7，滤除生成的 BaSO₄ 沉淀，滤液水浴浓缩至 1 ml，为供试品溶液。

③对照品溶液的制备　葡萄糖和鼠李糖对照品适量，以少量水溶解即得。展开剂：正丁醇 – 乙酸 – 水（4∶1∶5 上层或 4∶1∶1）。

用毛细管各吸取供试品和对照品溶液适量，点于滤纸上，用上述展开剂展开。展开剂吹干后，均匀喷以苯胺邻苯二甲酸盐试剂，105℃烘 5min，葡萄糖和鼠李糖均显棕色或棕红色斑点。

（3）光谱法鉴别

1）芦丁

UV（λ$_{max}$，nm）：357，258

IR（ν$_{max}$，KBr）：3422（broad，OH），1658（C＝O），1602，1502（benzene）

^{1}H-NMR（500 MHz，DMSO-d_6）中 δ：12.59（1H，s，5-OH），10.78（1H，s，7-OH），9.60（1H，s，4′-OH），9.12（1H，s，3′-OH），6.19（1H，d，J = 2.0 Hz，H-6），6.38（1H，d，J = 2.0 Hz，H-8），7.54（1H，dd，J = 8.0，2.2 Hz，H-6′），7.53（1H，s，H-2′），6.84（1H，d，J = 8.3 Hz，H-5′），5.34（1H，d，J = 7.4 Hz，H-1″），0.99（3H，d，J = 6.2 Hz，H-6‴）

2）槲皮素

UV（λ$_{max}$，nm）：357，258

IR（ν$_{max}$，KBr）：3600～2800（broad，OH），1640（C＝O），1500，1600（benzene）

^{1}H-NMR（400 MHz，DMSO-d_6，TMS）δ：12.50（1H，br.s，OH-5），7.66（1H，s，H-2′），7.53（1H，d，J = 8Hz，H-6′），6.87（1H，d，J = 8 Hz，H-5′），6.40（1H，s，H-8），6.18（1H，s，H-6）。

^{13}C-NMR（100MHz，DMSO-d_6，TMS）δ：175.6（C-4），163.8（C-7），160.5（C-5），156.0（C-9），147.5（C-4′），146.6（C-2），144.9（C-3′），135.5（C-3），121.8（C-1′），119.8（C-6′），115.5（C-5′），114.9（C-2′），102.8（C-10），98.1（C-6），93.3（C-8）

七、思考题

1. 影响芦丁提取的产率及质量的主要因素有哪些？

2. 如果芦丁酸水解反应未进行完全，产物会有何不同？

3. 用不同展开剂，或用不同类型的薄层色谱（或纸色谱）分析芦丁和槲皮素时，其结果有何不同？试用液相色谱的基本原理分析对各结构进行分析和说明。

扫码"练一练"

Experiment Ⅱ Extraction, Isolation and Identification of Rutin and Quercetin

1. Introduction

Huaihuami is *Sophora japonica* L. floral buds of Leguminosae family, used as a hemostatic. The main ingredient of the herb is Rutin.

Rutin, also called rutoside, quercetin-3-rutinoside and sophorin, is found in many plants, especially in *Sophora japonica* L. It is the glycoside between the flavonol quercetin and the disaccharide rutinose. It has the effect of reducing capillary permeability. It is used as an accessory drug to cure hypertension in clinical. In addition, Rutin has also the effect of holding back bleeding caused by radioactive rays.

Quercetin is the aglycone of rutin, and is found in citrus fruit, and many foods such as onions. Quercetin has demonstrated significant anti-inflammatory activity because of direct inhibition of several initial processes of inflammation.

2. Purposes

2.1 Learn the extraction, isolation method of flavonoids.

2.2 Familiar with the main chemical characteristics of flavonoids.

2.3 Learn the utilization of TLC and PC for the identification of flavone glycoside, aglucon and saccharide.

3. Principles

Rutin are pale yellow needles, the crystals contain 3 H_2O, m. p. 177 ~ 178℃. Rutin dissolves in boiling water (1 : 200), boiling methanol (1 : 7), cold methanol (1 : 100), boiling ethanol (1 : 30), and cold ethyl alcohol (1 : 300). It's slightly soluble in cold water (1 : 8000), ethyl acetate, acetone, practically insoluble in benzene, chloroform, ethyl ether and petroleum. Rutin has four phenyl hydroxyl group, it can dissolve in aqueous alkali and turn in yellow, but precipitate after acidification. Therefore, the "alkali extraction and acid precipitation" method can be used for extraction.

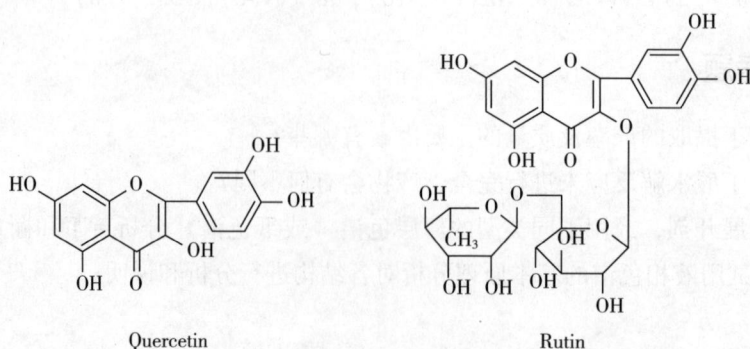

Quercetin   Rutin

Quercetin are yellow crystals, m. p. 313 ~ 314℃. It dissolves in boiling alcohol (1 : 23), cool

40

alcohol（1∶300）, glacial acetic acid, pyridine, ethyl acetate, and acetone et al. Quercetin practically insoluble in petroleum, benzene, ethyl ether, chloroform and water.

4. Apparatus and reagents

4. 1 Apparatus

Breakers（100 and 500ml）, flasks（100 and 150ml）, suction flask（500ml）, condenser, vacuum pump, UV-lamp, developing chamber for TLC, microcapillary（1mm）, Buchner funnel and stemmed funnel.

4. 2 Reagents

0. 4% sodium tetraborate, 2% H_2SO_4, limewater, HCl, Ba(OH)$_2$, AlCl$_3$, ethanol, methanol, poluamide TLC sheet, filter paper（5cm × 8cm）.

5. Developing solvents and references

5. 1 Developing Solvents

n-BuOH∶HAc∶H_2O（4∶1∶5 or 4∶1∶1）, EtOH∶H_2O（7∶3）.

5. 2 References

Rutin, Quercetin, Glucose, Rhamnose.

6. Procedures

6. 1 Isolation and purification of rutin

6. 1. 1 Extracting

In a 500ml flask place 20g of Huaihuami, add 250ml of 0. 4% sodium tetraborate. To the solution add limewater drop and keep the mixture stirring to adjust the pH 8, Heat to make the mixture boiled gently for 30 minutes, during this period, limewater was added to keep water and keep pH 8. Allow the solution to stand for about 10 minutes and cool it to room temperature, pour out the upper clear solution, filter to collect filtrate. Extract the crude medicine material repeatedly by the process described above, combine filtrate, adjust pH 2 ~ 3 with HCl, add 8 drops of EtOH, keep the solution over night, collect the crystals with suction on a Buchner funnel, wash the crystals 3 ~ 4 times with water, allow them to dry thoroughly in the air to get crude rutin. Weigh and calculate the yield.

6. 1. 2 Recrystallization

Dissolve 1g of crude Rutin in about 100ml water, make rutin dissolved as more as possible by warming on a water bath. Filter the hot solution to remove insoluble impurities. Concentrate the mother liquor to 20 ~ 30ml, allow the solution to cool and deposit crystals of rutin. Filter the cold solution to collect the crystals. Evaporate a half of water of the filtrate, and then make the solution cool to produce crystals again, filter and combine two parts of crystals, recrystallize with ethanol again to get purified rutin. Weigh and calculate the yield.

6. 2 Hydrolysis

In a 100ml round-bottomed flask provide with a reflux condenser, place 1g of Rutin and 50ml of 2% H_2SO_4. Add a boiling chip and boil gently for 1h. A yellow turbidity will appear gradually, which then turns into a fine needle. Cool the mixture to room temperature and filter the solution to obtain the crystals, i. e. crude quercetin. (Caution：20ml of filtrate need be reserved for the identification of saccharides.) Transfer the crude quercetin into a 100ml round-bottomed flask, add 50ml of 50% ethanol, reflux on a water bath until the solid has dissolved. Filter the hot solution, pour the filtrate into a 50ml conical flask, and allow it stand to yield a bright yellow precipitate, purified quercetin could be obtained with section, dry them under vacuum at 110℃ to give anhydrate quercetin, m. p. 313 ~ 314℃.

6.3 Treatment of sugar solution

Take 20 ml of the rutinic acid-retained filtrate and place it in a 50 ml beaker, and add about 2.6 g of $Ba(OH)_2$ fine powder in portions to neutralize the solution to pH 7, and filter out the formed $BaSO_4$ precipitate. Use filter paper to filter under normal pressure, and the filtrate is concentrated to 1-2 ml to obtain a concentrated sugar solution.

6.4 Identification

6.4.1 Identification of rutin and quercetin

6.4.1.1 Silica gel TLC

Samples：prepared rutin and quercetin, dissolved in ethanol.

References：rutin and quercetin for reference, dissolved in ethanol.

Developing solvent：BAW (4：1：5 upper layer or 4：1：1).

Appropriate amount of sample and reference solutions were applied with microcapillary, developpde by above solvents. Observe the spots either directly or exposing the sheet to UV light before and after the sheet was perfumed with $AlCl_3$ or NH_3.

6.4.1.2 Polyamide TLC

Samples：Prepared rutin and quercetin, dissolved in ethanol.

References：Rutin and quercetin for reference, dissolved in ethanol.

Developing Solvent：70% ethanol.

Appropriate amount of sample and reference solutions were applied with microcapillary, developed by above solvent. Observe the spots directly or exposing the sheet to UV light before and after the sheet was perfumed with $AlCl_3$ or NH_3.

6.4.2 Identification of saccharides

Filter paper：filter paper (5cm×8cm) .

Sample solution ：In a 50ml beaker place 20ml filtrate reserved (Section 6.2), add about 2.6g of $Ba(OH)_2$ in several times until the solution is neutralizd to pH 7. Filter it to remove $BaSO_4$ precipitate, concentrate the filtrate to about 1ml for the rest of saccharides.

Reference solution：glucose and rhamnose for reference, dissolved in water.

Developing solvent：BAW (4：1：5 upper layer or 4：1：1) .

Apply appropriate amount of sample and reference solutions with microcapillary, and develop the filter paper by above solvents. Aniline-*O*-phthalic acid reagent, heat the paper at 105 ℃ for about 5min. Both of glucose and rhamnose show brown to brown-red spots.

6.4.3 Identified by spectral data (see them in Chinese part.)

7. Questions

7.1 What are the main conditions related to the yield and quality of rutin?

7.2 What would happen if rutin was not hydrolyzed thoroughly?

7.3 Why do rutin and quercetin have different R_f value for different thin layer chromatographic system?

实验三　葛根中异黄酮类化合物的提取、分离和鉴定

一、简介

葛根来源于豆科常见的木质藤本植物野葛 *Pueraria lobata*（Willd.）Ohwi 的根，是我国重要的常用传统中药。其性甘、辛、凉，归脾、胃、肺经。具有退热解痉、生津止渴、升阳止泻、通经活络的功效，用于外感发热头痛、项背强痛、口渴、眩晕头痛、中风偏瘫等。葛根中含有多种异黄酮苷元及其苷类，葛根素和大豆苷元是其中两种主要活性成分。近代药理研究表明其具解热、消炎、抗菌、扩张冠脉血管、改善心肌缺血缺氧状态、改善脑血循环、降压等多种活性。

大豆苷元：白色结晶状粉末，m. p. 为 315～323℃，分子式 $C_{15}H_{10}O_4$，分子量为 254.24，溶于乙醚与乙醇。用于治疗高血压引起的心绞痛、头痛、眩晕，冠心病、妇女更年期综合症、骨质疏松等。

葛根素（8-β-D-葡萄吡喃糖-4′,7-二羟基异黄酮）：白色结晶（甲醇-乙酸），m. p. 187～189℃。$[\alpha]_D^{30}$ + 9.2°（c = 0.5，DMSO），分子式 $C_{21}H_{20}O_9$，分子量为 416.37。溶于水、甲醇、乙醇、吡啶，易溶于热水，难溶于苯、三氯甲烷、乙醚等，与醋酸镁反应显黄色，与醋酸铅反应呈黄色沉淀。具有扩张血管、降低血压、改善微循环、雌激素样作用和潜在的抗氧化作用。

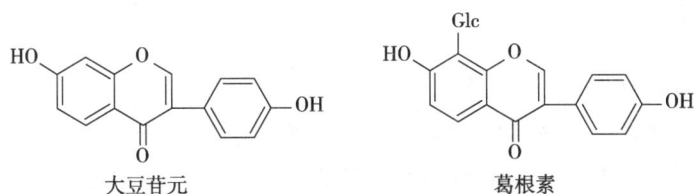

大豆苷元　　　　　　葛根素

二、目的

1. 学习从葛根中提取总异黄酮，以及利用硅胶、氧化铝、大孔树脂等柱色谱方法分离异黄酮类化合物的方法。

2. 学习运用 TLC 方法鉴别大豆苷元和葛根素。

三、原理

异黄酮及其苷是具有中等极性的成分，能用乙醇、甲醇等溶剂进行提取，并在乙酸乙酯、n-BuOH 与 H_2O 中进行分配。硅胶是常用的分离材料，根据其含水量可分为 I～V 级活度，一般 I～Ⅲ级为吸附分离原理，Ⅳ～V 级为分配分离原理。氧化铝可分为中性和碱性氧化铝，由于其具有碱性，分离酸性物质时需要避免或者注意。大孔吸附树脂是吸附性

和分子筛性原理相结合的分离材料，其吸附性是由范德华引力或氢键吸附共同作用的结果；分子筛则是由其本身多孔性结构的性质所决定。目前上述 3 种分离材料均广泛应用于天然产物的分离和富集，如多糖、黄酮（苷）、皂苷类等。在硅胶 TLC，异黄酮及其苷可以用 $FeCl_3 - K_3Fe(CN)_6$ 试剂显色，呈蓝色。

四、仪器与试剂

1. **仪器**　小层析缸（2 cm × 10 cm），分液漏斗（100 ml），旋转蒸发仪，硅胶 G 薄层板（微型），TLC 展开缸（微型），喷雾瓶，锥形瓶（50 ml），加热器或加热板。

2. **试剂**　硅胶（层析用），氧化铝（80～120 目），$CHCl_3$（A. R.），CH_3OH（A. R.），n-$BuOH$（A. R.），CH_3CH_2OH（A. R.），$FeCl_3$，$K_3Fe(CN)_6$，D101 大孔吸附树脂。

3. **对照品**　葛根素，大豆苷元。

五、操作

1. **总异黄酮的提取**　葛根粗粉 30 g，用 10 倍量 70% 乙醇于 500 ml 圆底烧瓶中回流提取 1 h，重复两遍。提取液过滤，旋转蒸发仪减压回收乙醇，得到的水浓缩液用等体积正丁醇萃取 3 遍，合并萃取液，减压除去正丁醇，得到粗品异黄酮混合物，干燥，称重，计算得率。

2. **总异黄酮的分离（根据实验条件选择）**

（1）葛根总异黄酮的氧化铝柱色谱　取总异黄酮样品 0.2 g，溶于少量水饱和的正丁醇，加于氧化铝柱（2.5 cm × 30 cm，空白氧化铝 30 g）的上端，用 100 ml 水饱和的正丁醇洗脱，收集流分，每 10 ml 一瓶，然后用 100 ml 正丁醇：吡啶（10：1）洗脱，旋转蒸发仪减压回收溶剂，得到各浓缩流分。用 TLC 方法检测各流分。

（2）葛根总异黄酮的硅胶柱色谱　取总异黄酮样品 0.2 g，溶于少量甲醇，加于硅胶柱（2.5 cm × 30 cm，200～300 目空白硅胶 30 g）的上端，进行低压硅胶柱色谱分离，用 300 ml 洗脱剂 $CHCl_3 - CH_3OH$（4：1）等度洗脱，收集流分，每 20 ml 一瓶，浓缩各流分得到不同流分，用 TLC 方法检测各流分。

（3）葛根总异黄酮的 D101 大孔树脂柱色谱　取总异黄酮样品 0.3 g，用适量水加热溶解，过滤，滤液加于预处理好的 D101 大孔树脂柱（2.5 cm × 30 cm，大孔树脂高 25 cm，湿法装柱）的上端，依次用 250 ml 蒸馏水，10%、30%、50%、70%、95% 乙醇-水洗脱，分别收集各不同溶剂洗脱馏分，浓缩各流分得到不同流分，用 TLC 方法检测各流分。

3. **异黄酮重结晶**

（1）葛根素的重结晶　取 0.1 g 葛根素粗品，用适量 90% 乙酸溶解，放置析晶，过滤，得葛根素结晶，干燥，称重，计算得率。

（2）大豆苷元的重结晶　取 0.1 g 大豆苷元粗品，溶解于适量 95% 乙醇，放置析晶，过滤，得大豆苷元结晶，干燥，称重，计算得率。

4. **异黄酮的结构鉴定**

（1）TLC 方法检测　样品用适量甲醇溶解，点于硅胶薄层板上，用 $CHCl_3 - CH_3OH$（4：1）为展开剂，$FeCl_3 - K_3Fe(CN)_6$ 喷雾显色，异黄酮斑点显蓝色，用大豆素、葛根素标准品进行对照。

（2）光谱方法鉴定

1）大豆苷元光谱数据

UV（λ_{max}，nm）：308，248

IR（ν_{max}^{KBr}，cm^{-1}）：3221～3020（broad，OH），1631（C＝O），1606，1517，1459

EI-MS（m/z）：254［M］$^+$

^{1}H-NMR（DMSO-d_6，300 MHz）δ ppm：8.22（1H，s，H-2），7.90（1H，d，$J=8.8$ Hz，H-5），7.32（1H，dd，$J=8.2$ Hz，H-2′,6′），6.87（1H，d，$J=2.2,8.8$ Hz，H-6），6.80（1H，d，$J=2.2$ Hz，H-8），6.75（1H，d，$J=8.2$ Hz，H-3′,5′）

^{13}C-NMR（DMSO-d_6，75 MHz）δ ppm：152.3（C-2），122.7（C-3），178.6（C-4），127.2（C-5），115.1（C-6），162.6（C-7），102.2（C-8），116.9（C-4a），157.6（C-8a），123.9（C-1′），130.0（C-2′），115.1（C-3′,5′），157.0（C-4′），130.0（C-6′）

2）葛根素光谱数据

UV（λ_{max}，nm）：305，250

IR（ν_{max}^{KBr}，cm^{-1}）：3351（broad，OH），1630（C＝O），1591，1514

EI-MS（m/z）：416［M］$^+$

^{1}H-NMR（DMSO-d_6，300 MHz）δ：8.34（1H，s，H-2），7.94（1H，d，$J=9.0$ Hz，H-5），7.39（1H，d，$J=8.9$ Hz，H-2′,6′），6.98（1H，d，$J=9.0$ Hz，H-6），6.80（1H，d，$J=8.9$ Hz，H-3′,5′），4.81（1H，d，$J=9.6$ Hz，H-1″）

^{13}C-NMR（DMSO-d_6，75 MHz）δ：154.5（C-2），125.7（C-3），178.4（C-4），128.2（C-5），116.7（C-6），163.0（C-7），113.3（C-8），118.6（C-4a），158.0（C-8a），124.2（C-1′），131.4（C-2′），116.3（C-3′,5′），158.8（C-4′），131.4（C-6′），82.8（C-1″），73.2（C-2″），75.8（C-3″），80.1（C-4″），71.8（C-5″），62.8（C-6″）

六、思考题

1. 叙述葛根异黄酮类化合物提取、分离的一般过程。

2. 迄今为止，从葛根中分离出了多少种异黄酮类化合物？

3. 葛根中异黄酮还有哪些提取分离方法？

Experiment Ⅲ Extraction，Isolation and Identification of Isoflavonoids in Pueraria Lobatea Radix

1. Introductions

Puerariae lobatea radix is the root of *Pueraria lobata*（Willd.）Ohwi, which is a perennial, woody climmber belongs to leguminosae. It is also an important Chinese traditional medicine. It possesses some activities such as abatement of fever, spasmolysis, producing saliva and slaking thirst. It has been used for the treatment of fever, apoplectic hemiplegia, dizziness, headache, thirst and spasm. Phytochemical investigation lead to the isolation of various isoflavonoids and its glycosides, but Daidzein and Puerarin are the main effective constituents. Modern pharmacological research indicated that this plant had many interesting activities including alleviating fever, anti-in-

扫码"练一练"

flammation, antibacterial, expanding coronary angiography, improving the state of myocardial ische-mia, hypoxia, blood circulation, and antihypertensive.

Daidzein: white crystalline powder, m. p. 315 ~ 323℃, molecular formula, $C_{15}H_{10}O_4$, molecular weight 254. 24. It can be dissovled in ethyl ether and ethanol. It has been used to treate angina, headache, dazziness induced by hypertension, coronary artery diseas, women climacteric syndrome or osteoporosis.

Puerarin (8-β-D-glucopyranoside-4', 7-dihydroxyl isoflavonoid): white crystal (MeOH-HAc), m. p. 187 ~ 189℃. $[\alpha]_D^{30}$ + 9. 2° (c = 0. 5, DMSO), molecular formula $C_{21}H_{20}O_9$, molecular weight 416. 37. It is dissolved in H_2O, MeOH, EtOH and pyridine, but difficultly dissolved in benzene, $CHCl_3$ and Et_2O. Its reaction with magnesium acetate displays yellow color, while yellow precipitate with Pb (Ac)$_2$ reaction. It was reported to expand blood vessel, lower blood pressure, improve microcirculation, and has estrogen-like effect and potential antioxidant activity.

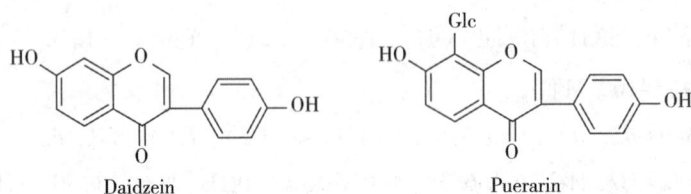

Daidzein   Puerarin

2. Purposes

2. 1 Students will learn the extraction and isolation methods of isoflavonoids from Pueraria lobatea radix by silica gel, Al_2O_3 and macroporous resin column chromatography.

2. 2 Students will learn to identify the structures of puerarin and daidzein by TLC method and spectroscopic method.

3. Principles

Isoflavonoids and its glycosides are constituents with moderate polarity, which can be extracted with alcoholic solvents, isolated by partition between EtOAc or n-BuOH and H_2O. Silica gel is the common materials used to isolate mixtures, which is divided into 5 activity grades based on their water content: grades Ⅰ – Ⅲ with absorption separation principles, grades Ⅳ – Ⅴ with partition separation principles. Aluminium oxide includes neutral and alkaline types. Because of its alkali properties, it is concerned that the isolation of acidic compounds need to be avoided or attention. However, macroporous resin is a kind of separation material with two principles combining molecular sieve and adsorption. Up to now, the above three materials are widely used in the separation and enrichment work of natural products, such as the polysacchairides, flavonoids (glycosides) and triterpenoids, etc. In silica-gel TLC test, isoflavonoids and its glycosides can react with $FeCl_3$-$K_3Fe(CN)_6$ and develop blue color.

4. Apparatus and reagents

4. 1 Apparatus

Small chromatography column (2 cm × 10 cm), Separation funnel (100 ml), Rotatory evaporator, Silica gel G TLC plates（micro size）, TLC development tank（mini type）, Spray reagent bottle, Conical flasks（50 ml）, Heater or hot plate.

4. 2 Reagents

Silica gel（column chromatography grade）, Alumina（80 ~ 120 mesh）, $CHCl_3$（A. R.）, MeOH（A. R.）, n-BuOH（A. R.）, $FeCl_3$, $K_3Fe(CN)_6$, D101 macroporous resin.

4. 3 References

Purarin, Daidzin.

5. Procedures

5. 1 Extraction of crude isoflavonoids

The 30 g powder of Puerariae lobetea radix is extracted with 10 volume ethanol（70%）in a 500 ml round-bottomed flask under reflux for 1 hour and repeated the operation for the second time. After removal of EtOH under reduced pressure, the aqueous concentrate was extracted with n-BuOH of same volume for three times. The extracts was combined and distilled the solvent under reduced pressure to afford crude isoflavonoids mixture. Dry, weigh and calculate the yield.

5. 2 Isolation of isoflavonoids（according to the experimental conditions）

5. 2. 1 Isolation of total isoflavones by Al_2O_3 column chromatography 0. 2 g crude isoflavonoids is dissolved in a small amount of n-butanol saturated with water, then subjected to Al_2O_3 column chromatography（2. 5 cm×30 cm, 30 g blank Al_2O_3）. The column was eluted with 100 ml of water-saturated n-butanol and then eluted with 100 ml of n-butanol pyridine（10∶1）, the speed of eluting was controlled at a rate of 10 ml/min. Collecting the eluent 10 ml per bottle, all the eluent were concentrated to dryness under a reduced pressure resulting in different dried fractions. Test all the fractions by TLC method.

5. 2. 2 Silica gel lower pressure column chromatography to isolate total isoflavonoids 0. 2 g crude isoflavonoids, dissolving in a small amount of MeOH, then separated on silica gel column chromatography under reduced pressure（2. 5 cm×30 cm, 30 g silica gel with 200 – 300 mesh）. The column was eluted with 300 ml $CHCl_3$ – MeOH（4∶1）, and collect each fraction per 20 ml eluent. All the eluent were concentrated to dry in vacuum leading to different fractions. Test all the fractions by TLC method.

5. 2. 3 Isolation of total isoflavones through D101 macroporous resin column chromatography 0. 3 g crude isoflavonoids is dissolved in a small amount of water and then filter. The filtrate is separated on pretreated D101 macroporous resin column chromatography（2. 5 cm × 30 cm, 25 cm height with D101 macroporous resin）. The column was eluted with 250 ml of distilled water, 10% EtOH、30% EtOH、50% EtOH、70% EtOH、95% EtOH, successively, then collect the corresponding eluent. All the eluent were concentrated to dry in vacuum to get different fractions. Test all the fractions by TLC method.

5. 3 Recrystallization of isoflavonoids

5. 3. 1 Recrystallization of purarin　Dissolve 0. 1 g crude purarin in 90% HAc, stand at room temperature to recrystallize, then filter to get purified purarin. Dry, weigh and calculate the yield.

5. 3. 2 Recrystallization of daidzin　Dissolve 0. 1 g crude purarin in 95% EtOH, stand at room

temperature to recrystallize, then filter to get purified daidzin. Dry, weigh and calculate the yield.

5. 4 Identification of structure of isoflavonoids

5. 4. 1 Identification by TLC method

Samples are dissolved in MeOH, then spot the solution on silica gel G plate, developing with $CHCl_3 - MeOH$ (4 : 1), sprayed with $FeCl_3 - K_3Fe$ (CN)$_6$ regent. Isoflavonoids appeared as blue spots. Compare them with standard compounds (purarin and daidzin).

5. 4. 2 Identification by Spectral Data (See them in the Chinese version).

6. Questions

6. 1 Describe the general process of extraction, isolation of the isoflavonoids of Pueraria lobata radix?

6. 2 How many kinds of isoflavonoids have been isolated and identified from Pueraria lobata radix?

6. 3 What are the other isolation methods of isoflavonoids of Pueraria lobata radix?

实验四　黄芩苷的提取、分离和鉴定

扫码"学一学"

一、简介

黄芩为唇形科植物黄芩 *Scutellaria baicalensis* Georgi 的干燥根，具有清热燥湿、泻火解毒、凉血安胎等作用，是我国常用中药材之一，应用历史悠久。黄芩苷（baicalin）是黄芩中主要有效成分，也是成药"双黄连注射剂""银黄制剂""三黄片"的主要成分，具有抑菌、清热、降压、解毒、镇静、抗炎、抗过敏、抗氧化等作用。近年来的研究发现，黄芩苷可抑制 HIV 病毒的感染和复制，从而成为一种治疗艾滋病的潜在药物。黄芩苷的化学名称为 5，6 – 二羟基黄酮 – 7 – O – β – D – 葡萄糖醛酸苷，别名为贝加灵，黄芩药材及大部分含黄芩的复方制剂均采用黄芩苷作为质量控制指标。

二、目的

1. 掌握酸性黄酮苷类成分的提取方法。
2. 熟悉大孔吸附树脂色谱法分离黄酮苷类成分。
3. 熟悉黄酮苷类化合物结构的检识、结构鉴定的一般程序和方法。
4. 了解正交设计实验法在优化化合物提取工艺中的应用。

三、原理

黄芩苷为黄色针状结晶（甲醇），熔点 223～225℃。可溶于热乙酸，难溶于甲醇、乙醇、丙酮，几乎不溶于水。在酸性条件下比较稳定，在稀 H_2SO_4（2%）水溶液中不会发生水解，但随着硫酸浓度增大、反应温度升高，则会发生水解，水解后生成其苷元——黄芩素（5，6，7 – 三羟基黄酮）。黄芩苷遇三氯化铁显绿色，遇醋酸铅生成橙色的沉淀。溶于碱及氨水初显黄色，久置则变为黑棕色。

因为黄芩苷结构中含有羧基，具有一定的酸性，故在植物中常以盐的形式存在，所以

提取黄芩苷时通常采用沸水提取法；再将提取液调成酸性，黄芩苷将在酸性水溶液中析出，再经过滤处理可与其他杂质分开。

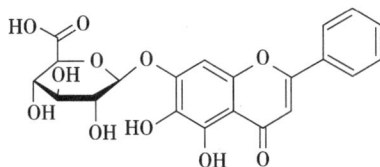

黄芩苷（Baicalin）

大孔吸附树脂是吸附性和分子筛性原理相结合的分离材料，它的吸附性是由于范德华引力和氢键共同作用的结果；分子筛性是由于其本身多孔性结构的性质所决定。现在已广泛应用于天然化合物的分离和富集工作中，如在多糖、黄酮（苷）、三萜类化合物的分离工作都有很好的应用。

四、仪器与试剂

1. 仪器 烧杯（100 ml、250 ml、500 ml），圆底烧瓶（500 ml），抽滤瓶（500 ml），冷凝管，层析柱（2 cm×30 cm），量筒（100 ml），布氏漏斗（中号），试管，玻棒，调温电热套，恒温水浴锅，旋转蒸发仪，循环水泵，电子天平。

2 试剂 镁粉，10% α-萘酚/乙醇溶液，2% 枸橼酸/甲醇溶液，2% $ZrOCl_2$/甲醇溶液，3% $FeCl_3$/乙醇溶液（加少量盐酸），40% NaOH，浓硫酸（分析纯），浓盐酸（化学纯），95% 乙醇，甲醇，乙酸乙酯（分析纯），D101 大孔吸附树脂，滤纸。

五、操作

1. 黄芩苷的提取和纯化

（1）提取（根据实验要求选择）

方法一：称取黄芩粗粉 30 g（不易过细，以免过滤时速度过慢），置 500 ml 烧杯中，加 8 倍量水，加热煮沸 1 h（随时补足因蒸发失去的水分）。然后过滤，滤渣中再加 6 倍量水，如上再提取第二次。合并两次提取液，在搅拌下向提取液中滴加浓盐酸调节 pH 1~2，放于 80℃ 水浴中保温 30 min，放冷析晶，然后进行抽滤，滤渣用水洗 3~4 次，自然干燥得粗品，称重。

方法二：称取黄芩粗粉 30 g（不易过细，以免过滤时速度过慢），置 500 ml 烧杯中，各实验小组按 L9（3^4）正交实验（见表 2-3、表 2-4）操作，合并提取液。在搅拌下向提取液中滴加浓盐酸调节 pH 1~2，放于 80℃ 水浴中保温 30min，放冷析晶，然后进行抽滤，滤渣用水洗 3~4 次，自然干燥得粗品，称重。以黄芩粗品的重量为指标，优化黄芩苷提取的最佳提取工艺条件。

表 2-3 正交试验因素水平表

水平	A 料/液比（g/ml）	B 提取次数	C 提取时间（min）
1	1:6	1	30
2	1:8	2	60
3	1:10	3	90

表 2 - 4　L9（3⁴）正交试验结果表

试验序号	列号				黄芩苷粗品重量（mg）
（分组）	A	B	C	D	
1	1	1	1	1	
2	1	2	2	2	
3	1	3	3	3	
4	2	1	2	3	
5	2	2	3	1	
6	2	3	1	2	
7	3	1	3	2	
8	3	2	1	3	
9	3	3	2	1	

（2）纯化（根据实验条件选择）

方法一：称取黄芩苷粗品 3 g 于 100 ml 烧杯中，加入 8 倍量水，搅拌均匀，用 40% NaOH 溶液调节至 pH 7，溶解，过滤，加等量乙醇（V/V），使黄芩苷成钠盐溶解，滤除杂质。滤液中滴加浓盐酸调节 pH 1~2，充分搅拌，50℃水浴中保温 90 min 使黄芩苷析出，滤出沉淀，以 10ml 50% 乙醇洗涤，干燥，得黄芩苷。再以 6~7 倍量 95% 乙醇洗涤，干燥，得精致黄芩苷，计算得率。

方法二：称取预处理好的 D101 大孔吸附树脂 20 g，湿法装柱。称取黄芩苷粗品 0.5 g 于 250 ml 烧杯中，加入 150 ml 蒸馏水，搅拌使其充分溶解，水溶液分别用 50 ml 乙酸乙酯（乙醚萃取效果好，但毒性大；用乙酸乙酯萃取时，有乳化现象，可将乳化层分离出，通过抽滤、静置，而达到分层的目的）萃取 3 次，保留水层（挥去乙酸乙酯）上柱，流速 2 ml/min；然后用 3 倍体积（约 120 ml）蒸馏水冲洗树脂柱，流速 3 ml/min；再用 3 倍体积的 50% 乙醇洗脱柱子，流速 3ml/min，收集洗脱液，减压浓缩，干燥，得精制黄芩苷，计算得率。

2. 黄芩苷的鉴定　称取黄芩苷 3 mg，加甲醇 9~10 ml 使其溶解，分成 4 份做下述实验。

（1）盐酸 - 镁粉反应　取上述溶液 0.5 ml 于白瓷板小孔中，加少许镁粉，振摇，再滴加 2 滴浓盐酸，观察并记录颜色变化。

（2）Molish 反应　取上述溶液 1~2 ml 于试管中，然后再加入等体积的 10% α - 萘酚/乙醇溶液，摇匀，沿管壁滴加浓盐酸，注意观察中部液面交界处颜色的变化，并记录实验结果。

（3）$ZrOCl_2$/枸橼酸反应　取上述溶液 1~2 ml 于试管中，然后滴加 2% $ZrOCl_2$/甲醇溶液，注意观察颜色变化情况，再继续向试管中加入 2% 枸橼酸/甲醇溶液，记录颜色变化情况。

（4）$FeCl_3$ 反应　取上述溶液 1~2 ml 于试管中，然后滴加 3% $FeCl_3$/乙醇溶液，观察并记录颜色变化情况。

3. 光谱法鉴别黄芩苷　黄芩苷的光谱数据如下。

UV（λ_{max}，nm）：314，278

IR（ν_{max}^{KBr}，cm^{-1}）：3416（broad，OH），1654（C＝O），1606，1580，1553，1493（benzene）1745，1076，897 为分子中的糖基吸收峰（1076 吸收峰来自于 C—O—C 糖苷键的伸缩振动，897 为 β-D 吡喃葡萄糖的特征吸收峰，1745 为—COOH 中 $\upsilon_{c=o}$ 引起的特征吸收峰）。

ESI-MS（m/z）：447 ［M + H］$^{+}$

^{1}H-NMR（DMSO-d_6,500MHz）δ：6. 82（1H，s，H-3），7. 00（1H，s，H-8），7. 94（1H，d，$J = 2. 0$Hz，H-2'），7. 53-7. 57（1H，m，H-4'），7. 94（1H，d，$J = 2. 0$Hz，H-6'），5. 23（1H，d，$J = 7. 3$Hz，H-1″），3. 42（1H，dd，H-2″），3. 37（1H，dd，H-3″），3. 46（1H，dd，H-4″），4. 07（1H，d，H-5″），12. 75（1H，br. s，5-OH），10. 38（1H，s，6-OH）

^{13}C-NMR（DMSO-d_6,125MHz）δ：164. 1（C-2），102. 6（C-3），182. 3（C-4），146. 9（C-5），130. 5（C-6），151. 0（C-7），93. 7（C-8），105. 9（C-4a），149. 0（C-8a），131. 8（C-1'），126. 3（C-2'），129. 0（C-3'），131. 6（C-4'），129. 0（C-5'），126. 3（C-6'），100. 1（C-1″），72. 8（C-2″），75. 2（C-3″），71. 3（C-4″），75. 5（C-5″），169. 9（C-6″）

六、思考题

1. 影响黄芩苷提取率的主要因素有哪些？

2. 用沸水提取法提取黄芩苷的原理是什么？

3. 用大孔树脂处理前为何要先用乙酸乙酯萃取，水相为何需挥去乙酸乙酯后才可用树脂处理？

扫码"练一练"

Experiment Ⅳ Extraction，Isolation and Identification of Baicalin

1. Introductions

Scutellariae radix is the dry root of *Scutellaria baicalensis* Georgi，known as Hollowgrass，Baicalin tea，Camellia roots，Kui baicalensis，Sub baicalensis，Article baicalensis，solani baicalensis and so on，which have the role of clearing heat and dampness，purging fire for removing toxin，removing heat from blood and tocolysis. It is one of the bulk of Chinese herbal medicines and has a long history application. Baicalin are the main active ingredient，but also the major components of medicines，such as " Shuanghuanglian injection"" Yinhuang agents"" sanhunag tabelts"，used as antibacterial，clearing heat，decompression，detoxication，sedation，anti-inflammation，anti-allergic，anti-oxidation. Especially in recent years，the study found that baicalin can prevent HIV infection and replication，thus becoming an effective drug for the treatment of AIDS. The chemical name is 5，6-dihydroxy-flavone-7-*O*-β-D-glucuronidase. Baicalin is used as quality control indicators in the *Scutellaria baicalensis* Georgi. herbal and most of the compound preparation.

2. Purposes

2. 1 Grasp the extraction method of acid flavonol glycoside.

2. 2 Familiar with the separation of flavonoid glycoside by macroporous resin chromatography.

2. 3 Familiar with the general procedures and methods of the structure identification of flavonoid glycosides.

2. 4 Understanding of orthogonal experimental design method in compounds extraction optimization.

3. Principles

Baicalin are yellow needle crystals (MeOH), melting point 223-225℃. Baicalin dissolves in hot acetic acid. It is insoluble in MeOH, EtOH, Me_2CO and hardly soluble in water. In relatively stable under acidic conditions, baicalin will not be hydrolysised in 2% H_2SO_4 aqueous solution. However, if increasing concentration of H_2SO_4 and the reaction temperature, the hydrolysis will be occurred, to generate baicalein. Baicalein (5,6,7-trihydroxyflavone) is the aglycones of baicalin. Baicalin can react with $FeCl_3$ and turn in green, when react with $Pb(Ac)_2$ and turn in orange precipitation. It can dissolve in aqueous alkali and turn in yellow, soon will become a black-brown.

Sincebaicalin has carboxyl and has a certain acidic, in plants it often exists in the form of salt, so the boiling water is often used to extract it. Adjust the extract to acidity, baicalin will be separated out in acidic solution, and be separated from other impurities by the filters.

Macroporous resin is a kind of separation materials, which has the principle of combining molecular sieve with adsorption. It is now widely used in the separation and enrichment work of natural products, such as the polysacchairides, flavonoids (glycosides) and triterpenoids, etc.

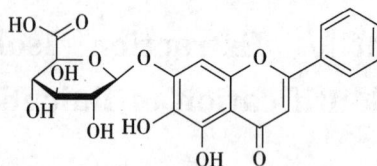

Baicalin

4. Apparatus and reagents

4. 1 Apparatus

Beakers (100, 250 and 500 ml), flasks (500 ml), suction flask (500 ml), condenser, chromatography column (2 cm × 30 cm), graduated flask (100 ml), buchner funnel (middle size), test tubes, glass rod, electric jacket, thermostat water bath, rotary evaporator, vacuum pump, electronic balance.

4. 2 Reagents

Mg powder, 10% α-naphthol/EtOH solution, 2% citric acid/MeOH solution, 2% $ZrOCl_2$/MeOH solution, 3% $FeCl_3$/EtOH solution (bit HCl), 40% NaOH, H_2SO_4 (AR), HCl (CP), 95% EtOH, MeOH, EtOAc (AR), D101 macroporous resin, filter paper.

5. Procedures

5. 1 Extraction and rurification of baicalin

5. 1. 1 Extraction (according to the experiment requires)

Method I : In a 500 ml breaker place 30g of Huangqin coarse powder, add 8-fold water, heat to boil 1 hour (complement the evaporation of water at any time), then filter and add 6-fold water into filter residue as the second extraction. Merge the two extracts, add HCl to the solution and keep the mixture stirring to adjust the pH from 1 to 2. Then put it in 80℃ water bath for 30 minutes, keep the solution cool and crystal precipitation, filter the crystals with a buchner funnel, wash the crystals 3~4 times with water, allow them to dry thoroughly in the air to get crude baicalin and weigh.

Method Ⅱ: In a 500 ml breaker place 30 g of huangqin coarse powder, the experimental group operates according to the L9（3⁴）orthogonal test（table 2-3, table 2-4）. Merge the extracts, add HCl to the solution and keep the mixture stirring to adjust the pH from 1 to 2. Then put it in 80℃ in a water bath for 30 minutes, keep the solution cool and crystal precipitation, filter the crystals with a Buchner funnel, wash the crystals 3~4 times with water, allow them to dry thoroughly in the air to get crude Baicalin and weigh. Optimize the extraction conditions of baicalin with the weight of crude Baicalin as indicators,

Table 2 – 3   Orthogonal test factor level table

Level	A Material/liquid ratio（g/ml）	B Extraction times	C Extraction time（min）
1	1 : 6	1	30
2	1 : 8	2	60
3	1 : 10	3	90

Table 2 – 4   Results table of L9（3⁴）orthogonal test

Test serial number	No. row				Weight of Baicalin Crude（mg）
	A	B	C	D	
1	1	1	1	1	
2	1	2	2	2	
3	1	3	3	3	
4	2	1	2	3	
5	2	2	3	1	
6	2	3	1	2	
7	3	1	3	2	
8	3	2	1	3	
9	3	3	2	1	

5.1.2 Purification（according to the experimental conditions）

Method one: Dissolve 3 g of crudeBaicalin in about 8-fold of water in a 100 ml beaker, mix and add 40% NaOH solution to adjust the pH 7, make Baicalin dissolved as more as possible. Add equivalence EtOH and filter the solution to remove insoluble impurities. Add HCl by drop to the filtrate and keep the mixture stirring to adjust the pH from 1 to 2. Then put it in 50℃ water bath for 90 minutes, make Baicalin crystal precipitation, filter the crystals with a Buchner funnel, wash the crystals with 10 ml 50% EtOH. Then wash the crystals with 6 or 7-fold 95% EtOH, dry to get purified Baicalin. Weigh and calculate the yield.

Method two: Put 20 g pretreated D101 macroporous resin into the columns. Dissolve 0.5 g crude Baicalin in about 150 ml of distilled water in a 250 ml beaker, make Baicalin dissolved as more as possible by mixture. Extract the water solution with 50 ml EtOAc for 3 times, then put the water layer into the columns. Keep the velocity at 2 ml/min, then flush the resin column with 3BV (about 120 ml) distilled water at the velocity of 3 ml/min. Finally flush the resin column with 3BV (about 120 ml) 50% EtOH at the velocity of 3 ml/min. Combine the 50% EtOH eluent and concentrate it under vacuum condition, dry to get purified Baicalin. Weigh and calculate the yield.

5. 2 Identification of baicalin

Dissolve 3mg baicalinin with 9 ~ 10ml MeOH, then divide it into 4 parts to do the following test.

5. 2. 1 HCl-Mg powder reaction   Put 0. 5 ml the above solution into a test tube, add little Mg powder, then add 2 drops HCl, observe and record the color changes.

5. 2. 2 Molish reaction   Put 1 ~ 2 ml the above solution into a test tube, add equal volume 10% α-naphthol/EtOH solution and shake, then add HCl along the wall, observe the color changes at the surface at the junction of the central, and record the test results.

5. 2. 3 ZrOCl$_2$/citric acid reaction   Put 1 ~ 2 ml the above solution into a test tube, add 2% ZrOCl$_2$/MeOH solution, observe the color changes; then add 2% citric acid/MeOH solution into the test tube, record the color changes.

5. 2. 4 FeCl$_3$ reaction   Put 1-2 ml the above solution into a test tube, add 3% FeCl$_3$/MeOH solution, observe and record the color changes.

5. 3. Spectral datas of Baicalin (See them in the Chinese Part.)

6. Questions

6. 1 What are the main factors that influence the rate of extraction of Baicalin?

6. 2 What is the principle of extracting Baicalin with boiling water?

6. 3 Why extract the water solution with EtOAc before treat with macroporous resin? Why volatilize the EtOAc in the water solution before treat with macroporous resin?

实验五　苦参碱和氧化苦参碱的提取、分离和鉴定

一、简介

中药苦参是豆科槐属植物苦参 *Sophora flavescens* Ait. 的干燥根，味苦，性寒，具有清热燥湿，杀虫等作用。苦参主要含有生物碱、黄酮等化学成分。苦参碱和氧化苦参碱为苦参代表性生物碱，药理实验和临床用药证明二者具有多种生理活性，临床上主要用于治疗癌症、病毒性肝炎、病毒性心肌炎及某些皮肤疾患。

二、目的

1. 掌握从苦参中提取生物碱的方法。
2. 掌握用硅胶柱色谱技术分离生物碱的方法。
3. 掌握通过 TLC 及波谱学方法鉴定苦参碱和氧化苦参碱结构的方法。

扫码"学一学"

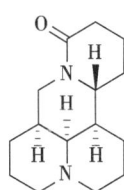 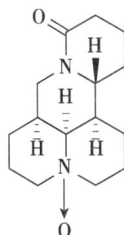

苦参碱　　　　　　　氧化苦参碱

三、原理

苦参碱是具有喹诺里西啶类结构母核的叔胺碱，有四种晶体类型：α-苦参碱（针晶或柱晶），m. p. 76℃；β-苦参碱（六边形），m. p. 87℃；γ-苦参碱（斜柱体），m. p. 223℃，δ-苦参碱（柱晶），m. p. 84℃。最常见的结晶形态是 α-苦参碱，溶于水、苯、乙醚、三氯甲烷、乙醇等溶剂，而几乎不溶于石油醚。氯化苦参碱是苦参碱的 N-氧化物，它溶于水、三氯甲烷、丙酮和乙醇而几乎不溶于乙醚。

苦参碱和氧化苦参碱遇酸成盐，故溶于稀酸水。将苦参生物碱的酸水提取液通过阳离子交换树脂柱进行交换，然后阳离子交换树脂用浓氨水碱化，再用三氯甲烷提取得到生物碱粗品。通过低压硅胶柱色谱，用 $CHCl_3$、CH_3OH 混和溶剂洗脱，浓缩各洗脱流分，得到苦参碱和氧化苦参碱。

四、仪器与试剂

1. **仪器**　色谱柱（小：2 cm × 10 cm；大：5 cm × 30 cm），分液漏斗（100 ml），旋转蒸发仪，硅胶 G 薄层色谱板（载玻片），薄层色谱展开缸（小型），喷雾瓶，圆底烧瓶（50ml），加热器或加热板，氮气钢瓶。

2. **试剂**　阳离子交换树脂（Amberlite IRC – 50），柱色谱用硅胶、锌粉、三氯甲烷（A. R.）、甲醇（A. R.）、丙醇（A. R.）、乙醇（A. R.）、碘化铋钾试剂，盐酸（A. R.）、浓氨水。

五、操作

1. **苦参碱和氧化苦参碱的提取、分离和鉴别**　苦参饮片 300 g 用 3 L 稀酸水提取两次，合并酸水提取液，使其通过阳离子交换树脂柱。树脂用蒸馏水洗涤几次，干燥后，加入 15% 的浓氨水以游离生物碱。将树脂转入索氏提取器，用 200 ml $CHCl_3$ 提取生物碱。

得到的生物碱混合物上低压硅胶柱色谱，用不同比例的 $CHCl_3$ – MeOH（100∶1，50∶1，20∶1）作为洗脱剂。用 TLC 法检测，将各流分分别点样于硅胶板上，用 $CHCl_3$ – CH_3OH（9∶1）（氨气饱和）作为展开剂，用苦参碱和氧化苦参碱标准品作对照，改良碘化铋钾试剂显色，比较 R_f 值，得到苦参碱和氧化苦参碱。

2. **氧化苦参碱的还原**　取氧化苦参碱粗品 1.0 g，溶于 15 ml 10% 盐酸水溶液中，放入 1.0 g 锌粉，室温放置，不时摇动，放置 24 h 后过滤，溶液调 pH 至 9～10，用 500 ml 乙醚分多次萃取，合并乙醚溶液，无水硫酸钠干燥过夜。回收乙醚得淡黄色黏稠液体（放置于冰箱中，得浅黄色固体），石油醚重结晶后得白色晶体。测熔点。

扫码"看一看"

3. 苦参碱和氧化苦参碱的结构鉴定

（1）薄层色谱法

样品：苦参碱标准品，氧化苦参碱标准品，苦参碱（自制），氧化苦参碱（自制）

溶剂系统：$CHCl_3 : CH_3OH = 8 : 2$，氨气饱和

TLC 板：硅胶 G 薄层色谱板

显色剂：改良碘化铋钾试剂

（2）光谱法鉴别

1）苦参碱的光谱数据

UV（λ_{max}，nm）：205

IR（ν_{max}，KBr，cm^{-1}）：2920，2840（CH），2790，2750（Bohlmann band），1640，1620，1460

EI-MS（m/z）：248［M］$^+$（100%），247［M-H］$^-$

^{1}H-NMR（$CDCl_3$，500 MHz）δ：3.82（1H，dt，$J = 9.6$，6.0 Hz，H-11），2.43（1H，dt，$J = 17.4$，4.2 Hz，H-14b），2.25（1H，m，H-14b），4.40（1H，dd，$J = 12.6$，4.2 Hz，H-17a），3.05（1H，t，$J = 12.6$ Hz，H-17b）

^{13}C-NMR（$CDCl_3$，125 MHz）δ：57.3（C-2），21.1（C-3），27.1（C-4），35.3（C-5），63.8（C-6），41.4（C-7），26.4（C-8），20.8（C-9），57.2（C-10），53.1（C-11），27.7（C-12），19.0（C-13），32.8（C-14），169.3（C-15），43.2（C-17）

2）氧化苦参碱的光谱数据

UV（λ_{max}，nm）：202

IR（ν_{max}，KBr，cm^{-1}）：3470，2940，1615（C=O），1470，1440，1420

EI-MS（m/z）：264［M］$^+$，247［M—OH］（100%），205

^{1}H-NMR（$CDCl_3$，500MHz）δ：5.09（1H，dt，$J = 10.2$，6.0 Hz，H-11），2.45（1H，m，H-14a），2.22（1H，m，H-14b），4.42（1H，dd，$J = 12.0$，5.4 Hz，H-17a），4.17（1H，t，$J = 12.6$ Hz，H-17b）

^{13}C-NMR（$CDCl_3$，125MHz）δ：69.1（C-2），17.1（C-3），26.1（C-4），34.5（C-5），67.1（C-6），42.6（C-7），24.6（C-8），17.2（C-9），69.5（C-10），52.9（C-11），28.5（C-12），18.6（C-13），32.9（C-14），170.0（C-15），41.7（C-17）

六、思考题

1. 叙述苦参中生物碱提取、分离的一般方法。

2. 叙述硅胶色谱柱的几种装柱方法。

3. 槐属植物中已分离、鉴定的生物碱有几种？

Experiment Ⅴ Extraction, Isolation and Identification of Matrine and Oxymatrine

1. Introduction

Traditional Chinese Medicines "Kushen" is the dry roots of the plants of *Sophora flavescens*

Ait. which belongs to family Leguninosae. There are two major kinds of chemical constituents, alkaloids and flavanoids, in Kushen. Matrine and oxymatrine are the two principle alkaloid components in the root of *S. flavescens* Ait. An intensive investigation into the pharmacology and clinical applications of these alkaloids has been continued for the past decades and remains one of the hot focuses in Chinese medical research. The main clinical applications are the treatment of cancer, viral hepatitis, cardiac diseases and some skin diseases.

2. Purpose

2. 1 Students will learn the extraction methods of alkaloids from the plants of Sophora flavescens and the of their structures.

2. 2 Students will learn the isolation methods of alkaloids by silica gel column chromatography.

2. 3 Students will learn the identification methods of Matrine and Oxymatrine by TLC and spectra.

3. Principle

Matrine, the main active constituent in the material medica *Sophora flavescens* Ait. , *S. alopecudoides* L, *S. subprostrata* Chun et T. Chen, is a tertiary amine alkaloid with the mother structure classified into tetracycloquinolizindine. There are four kinds of its crystals: α-matrine (needles or cylindrical crystal), m. p. 76℃; β-matrin (hexagonal crystal), m. p. 87℃; γ-matrine (liquid), m. p. 223℃, δ-matrine (cylindrical crystal), m. p. 84℃. The most frequently-used type is α-matrine, which is soluble in water, benzene, ether, chloroform, ethanol but slightly in petroleum ether. Oxymatrine is the *N*-oxide of Matrine. It dissolves in water, chloroform, acetone and ethanol but slightly in ether.

Both of matrine and oxymatrine can be dissolved in dilute acidic solution as salts. Let the total alkaloid salts solution of Kushen through a column of Amberlite (H^+ type), they will be absorbed on it. The cation exchange resin is made basic with concentrated ammonia and the alkaloid mixture is extracted with $CHCl_3$. The alkaloid mixture is chromatographed on silica gel column, eluting with different proportions of $CHCl_3$ and CH_3OH, then concentrate the elution to obtain matrine and oxymatrine.

4. Main apparatus and reagents

4. 1 Apparatus

Chromatography column (Small: 2 cm × 10 cm; big: 5 cm × 30 cm), Separation funnel (100 ml), Rotatory evaporator, Silica gel G TLC plates (micro size), TLC development tank (mini type), Spray reagent bottle, Conical flasks (50 ml), Heater or hot plate, Nitrogen gas steel tank

4. 2 Reagents

Amberlite IRC-50, Silica gel (column chromatography grade), Zn powder, $CHCl_3$(A. R.), CH_3OH(A. R.), Acetone(A. R.), C_2H_5OH(A. R.), Dragendorff's reagent, HCl(A. R.), concentrate ammonia.

5. Procedures

5. 1 Extraction，separation，and identification of matrine and oxymatrine

Material of Kushen （300 g） is extracted twice with 3 L dilute acidic water for one day at room temperature. The combined water extract is passed through a column of Amberlite IRC − 50. 15% concentrate ammonia is added to the cation exchange resin to free the absorbed alkaloids.

Putting the resin into a shoxlet extracter，using 200 ml $CHCl_3$ to extract the alkaloids. The obtained mixture of alkaloids is chromatographed on silica gel column under low pressure， using different proportions of $CHCl_3$ − MeOH （100 : 1，50 : 1，20 : 1） as eluents. Detecting the eluting solutions with TLC method. Spotting the solution on to silica gel G plate，developing with $CHCl_3$ − CH_3OH （9 : 1）（The tank is filled with ammonia gas）. Spraying the Dragendorff reagent. Comparing the value of R_f with standard Matrine and Oxymatrine.

5. 2 Reduction of oxymatrine

Get 1. 0g of crude oxymatrine dissolved in 15 ml of hydrochloric acid aqueous with the percebtage of 10%，put in 1. 0g of powder Zn at room temperature，shake it at intervals，then filter after 24h. the solution was modulated the pH 9 ~ 10，the extrate with 200ml of ether for many times. Combining the ether，add in dessicant of anhydrous sodium sulfate and put overnight. Distilling out the ether，the remine was light yellowish mucous liquid （place it in refrigerater，can get light yellowish solid），with crystals can emerge by recrystallizing in petroleum ether，detecting the melting point.

5. 3 Identification of structures of Matrine and Oxymatrine

5. 3. 1 Identification by TLC method

Samples：Standard Matrine, Standard Oxymatrine, Prepared Matrine, Prepared Oxymatrine

Developing solvent：$CHCl_3$: CH_3OH = 8 : 2，the tank was saturated with ammonia gas.

Detecting reagent：Modified Dragendorff's reagent.

5. 3. 2 Identified by Spectral data （See them in Chinese version）

6. Questions

6. 1 Generally describe the process of extracting and isolating of alkaloids from Kushen.

6. 2 Describe the different methods to make the silica gel column chromatography.

6. 3 How many kinds of alkaloids have been isolated and identified from the plants of Sophora ?

实验六　掌叶防己碱的提取、分离及延胡索乙素的制备

一、简介

防己科植物黄藤（Daemonorops margaritae）中主要含有掌叶防己碱（巴马汀），此外还有药根碱、非洲防己碱、黄藤素甲、黄藤素乙、黄藤内酯等。

掌叶防己碱是季铵生物碱，溶于水、乙醇，几乎不溶于三氯甲烷、乙醚等溶剂，主要具有抗菌作用。掌叶防己碱盐酸盐即氯化巴马汀为黄色针状结晶，m. p. 206℃（分解），经

氢化后即得延胡索乙素（四氢巴马汀），m. p. 146～148℃。黄藤中掌叶防己碱含量高达4%，而延胡索乙素在延胡索中含量仅为万分之几，所以黄藤为生产延胡索乙素提供了丰富的资源。

二、目的

1. 掌握渗漉提取的方法。
2. 得到巴马汀。
3. 学习巴马汀的氢化方法。
4. 学习生物碱的定性鉴别方法。
5. 学习生物碱的 TLC 鉴别方法。

三、原理

黄藤中巴马汀（掌叶防己碱，Palmatine）的含量为 4%，是季铵型生物碱，可溶于水、甲醇、乙醇中，其盐酸盐的溶解度低，有机酸盐的溶解度高，因此，以 1% 的醋酸溶液用渗漉法提取巴马汀，所得提取液应用盐析的方法，使巴马汀在水中溶解度降低而沉淀出来。氯化巴马汀经四氢硼钠氢化得到延胡索乙素。

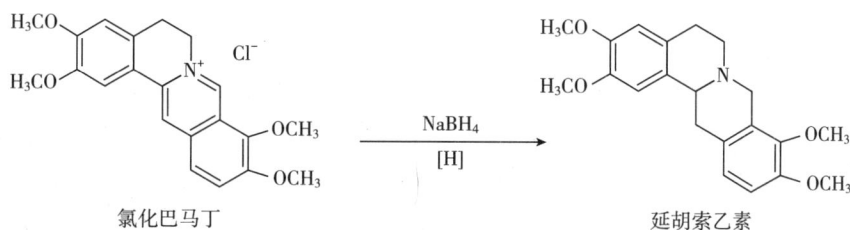

氯化巴马丁　　　　　　　　　　　　　　延胡索乙素

四、仪器与试剂

1. **仪器**　烧杯（100 ml，1000 ml），抽滤瓶，渗漉筒，层析缸，100 ml 锥形瓶，喷瓶，氨缸。

2. **试剂**　1% 乙酸，氯化钠，生物碱沉淀试剂（碘化铋钾、碘化汞钾、碘－碘化钾、硅钨酸、苦味酸）。

3. **展开剂**　三氯甲烷：甲醇（7:3）。

4. **对照品**　氯化巴马汀，延胡索乙素。

五、操作

1. **提取**　称取黄藤粉末 40g，置 100 ml 烧杯中，加 1% 乙酸 25 ml，搅拌 15min。置润湿好的粉末于玻璃渗漉筒中，加 1% 乙酸 500 ml 渗漉，调节渗漉速度为每秒 1～2 滴。

收集 10 ml 渗漉液，分装于 5 支试管中，分别滴加生物碱沉淀试剂碘化铋钾、碘化汞钾、碘－碘化钾、硅钨酸和苦味酸，检查药材中是否有生物碱。

剩余渗漉液按 10%（W/V）加入 NaCl，加入 40% NaOH 至 pH 10，放置过夜使析出固体，小心倾倒上清液，抽滤，干燥得粗巴马汀。称重，计算得率。

2. **巴马汀的精制**　置粗巴马汀于圆底烧瓶中，加 80% 乙醇 30ml 回流 5 min，加热溶解，趁热抽滤，滤渣再加 20ml 80% 乙醇加热溶解，趁热抽滤。合并滤液于 100ml 三角瓶，加 6 mol/L HCl 调至 pH 2，放置过夜析晶，抽滤，干燥，得氯化巴马汀。称重，计算得率。

3. 氢化 称取 1g 氯化巴马汀，置 100ml 三角瓶中，加 50% 甲醇 30ml 加热溶解，加入 0.8～1.0g 四氢硼钠，边加边搅拌至无气泡产生，再加入 6 mol/L HCl 调 pH 2 至无气泡产生。加入 NH₄OH 调至 pH 9，放置约 15 min，抽滤。滤渣加 95% 乙醇，回流溶解，趁热抽滤，滤液加 2～3 倍量的水，摇匀静置使析出沉淀，抽滤，取滤饼，干燥，得延胡索乙素。称重，计算得率。

4. 巴马汀和延胡索乙素的薄层鉴定

（1）样品溶液 自制巴马汀和延胡索乙素少量，以适量乙醇溶解。

（2）对照品溶液 巴马汀和延胡索乙素适量，以适量乙醇溶解。

（3）展开剂 三氯甲烷 – 甲醇（7∶3）

用毛细管各吸取样品和对照品溶液适量，点于硅胶 G 薄层板上，置硅胶板于氨缸中放置 5 min。用上述展开剂展开。展开剂吹干后，在紫外光下观察色斑，再喷碘化铋钾显色剂观察。

5. 巴马汀和延胡索乙素的光谱法鉴别

（1）巴马汀光谱数据

UV（λ_{max}，nm）：267，265，349，431

IR（ν_{max}，KBr）：3419（N-H），1606，1517（芳环）

^{1}H-NMR（CDCl₃，300MHz）δ：7.71，（1H，s，H-1），7.06（1H，s，H-4），4.99（1H，m，H-5），3.23（1H，m，H-6），9.91（1H，s，H-8），8.17（1H，d，J=9.2Hz，H-11），8.06（1H，d，J=9.15Hz，H-12），9.19（1H，s，H-14），3.86，3.93，4.05，4.10，（12H，s，OCH₃×4）。

^{13}C-NMR（CDCl₃，75MHz）δ：108.9（C1），148.8（C2），150.2（C3），111.3（C4），128.5（C4a），26.1（C5），62.0（C6），145.4（C8），119.0（C8a），151.5（C9），143.7（C10），123.6（C11），120.1（C12），133.2（C12a），126.7（C13），137.6（C14），121.4（C14a），55.4，55.9，56.4，57.1（OCH₃×4）。

（2）延胡索乙素光谱数据

UV（λ_{max}，nm）：213，281。

IR（ν_{max}，KBr）：3427（N-H），1511，1610（芳环）。

^{1}H-NMR（CDCl₃，300MHz）δ：6.73（1H，s，H-1），6.62（1H，s，H-4），2.64（1H，m，H-5），3.18（1H，m，H-6），4.26（1H，m，H-8a），3.51（1H，m，H-8b），6.89（1H，d，J=8Hz，H-11），6.80（1H，d，J=8Hz，H-12），3.29（1H，m，H-14a），2.83（1H，m，H-14b），3.88，3.87，3.85，3.85，（12H，s，OCH₃×4）。

^{13}C-NMR（CDCl₃，75MHz）δ：108.7（C1），147.4（C2），147.5（C3），111.0（C4），127.8（C4a），29.1（C5），51.5（C6），54.0（C8），126.8（C8a），150.2（C9），145.1（C10），123.8（C11），111.4（C12），128.7（C12a），36.3（C13），60.1（C14），129.7（C14a），55.8，55.9，59.3，56.1（OCH₃×4）。

六、注意事项

1. 提取之前，加入少量乙酸溶液使药材充分膨胀非常重要，这样可以避免药材粉末在渗漉筒中膨胀而使提取液流出困难。

2. 提取前将 2 层湿纱布铺在渗漉筒底端孔中，将粉末均匀倒入筒中，上面再铺一层滤纸。

3. 将渗漉筒阀门打开，加满提取液，关闭阀门，浸泡药材粉末 10 min，然后开始提取。

4. 加入的氯化钠（盐析）的重量为提取液体积的 10% 。

七、思考题

1. 可用什么方法提取黄藤中生物碱？请设计提取流程。

2. 氯化巴马汀氢化成延胡索乙素后，为什么颜色由黄变成无色？

3. 避免生物碱在硅胶板上拖尾的方法有哪些？

扫码"练一练"

Experiment Ⅵ　Extraction, Isolation and Hydrogenation of Palmatine and Preparation of Tetrahydropalmatine

1. Introduction

Palmatine is a quaternized alkaloid and the main alkaloids in *daemonorops margaritae* in addition to jatrorrhizine, columbamine, fibranine, fibraminine and fibralaetone.

Palmatine can be dissolved in water, ethanol, but practically insoluble in chloroform and ethyl ether. Palmatine hydrochloride or chloride palmatine is a yellow needle crystal and the melting point is 206℃ (decomposition), which can be turned into tetrahydropalmatine (corydalis B, white crystal, m. p. 146～148℃). The content of palmatine in *daemonorops margaritae* is about 4%, while tetrahydropalmatine, a drug used for a analgesic in clinic, has only a few content. Thus, we can obtain tetrahydropalmatine from palmatine by the reaction of hydrogenation.

2. Purpose

（1）Learn the extraction method of percolation.

（2）To obtain palmatine.

（3）Learn the hydrogenation method of palmatine

（4）Learn the qualitative identification method of alkaloid.

（5）Learn how to identify alkaloids by TLC.

3. Principles

The content of palmatine in *daemonorops margaritae* is about 4%. The quaternary alkaloids can be dissolved in water, alcohol and methyl alcohol, and its hydrochloride has lower solubility in the kinds of solvents but higher solubility of organic salts. Therefore, we can extract palmatine with 1% acetic acid by percolation and precipitate it out by adding inorganic salt. Chloride palmatine can be turned into tetrahydropalmatine by hydrogenation with $NaBH_4$ easily.

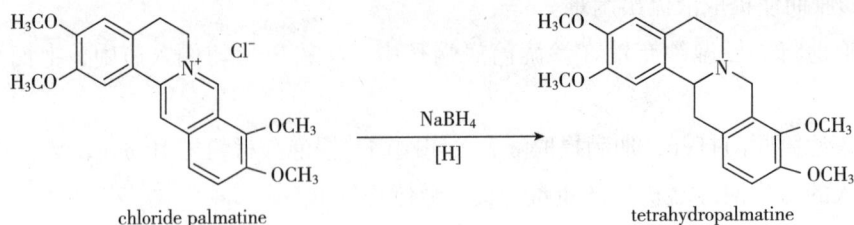

chloride palmatine   tetrahydropalmatine

4. Apparatus and reagents

4. 1 Apparatus

100ml, 1000ml beaks, suction filtering flask, percolation tube, TLC development tank, 100ml conical flasks, spray reagent bottle, ammonia tank.

4. 2 Reagents

1% acetic acid, sodium chloride, alkaloids precipitation reagent (Dragendorff, Mayer, Wagner, Silicowolframic acid, TrinitropHenol).

4. 3 Developing solvents.

$CHCl_3$: MeOH (7∶3)

4. 4 Reference Solution

Palmatine, tetrahydropalmatine.

5 Procedures

5. 1 Extracting method

Weigh out the powder of the plant 40g, transfer it to a 100 ml beak, add 25 ml of 1% acetic acid and stir it for 15 minutes to make the full expansion of medicinal herbs. Then transfer it to a glass percolation tube, add about 500ml of 1% acetic acid, regulating valve to make the flow rate at 1-2 drips/second.

Collecting 10 ml extracted solution and divided it to 5 test tubes, add the test reagent such as dragendorff, mayer, wagner, silicowolframic acid and trinitrophenol respectively to make sure if there are alkaloids in the plant.

Collecting extracted solution, add NaCl in accordance with the 10% (W/V) ratio to percolation liquid, then adjust the solution to pH 10 with 40% NaOH, keep the solution over night. Last, pour out the upper clear solution, filter and dry the residue in oven to obtain crude palmatine. Weigh and calculate the yield.

5. 2 Recrystallization

The crude palmatine mentioned above was refluxed for 15 minutes with 30 ml 80% ethanol, immediate filtration. The residue was refluxed with 20 ml 80% ethanol, filter, combine the filtrate, adjust the solution to pH 2 with 6 mol/L HCl, keep the solution over night. Filter and dry to obtain chloride palmatine. Weigh and calculate the yield.

5. 3 Hydrogenation

Dissolve 1g chloride palmatine with 30 ml 50% MeOH in a conical flask, add 0. 8-1. 0g NaBH₄ with stirring until no bubbles in the solution. Then adjust the pH to 2 with 6 mol/L HCl until no bubbles in it, adjust the solution to pH 9 with NH_4OH, stand for about 15 minutes, filter. The residue was refluxed with 95% ethanol, immediate filtration, add 2 to 3 times the amount of water, stand for about 20 minutes, filter and dry to obtain tetrahydropalmatine. Weigh and calculate the yield.

5. 4 TLC identification

Samples：Prepared Palmatine and tetrahydropalmatine, dissolved in ethanol.

Reference solution：Palmatine and tetrahydropalmatine, dissolved in ethanol.

Developing Solvent：$CHCl_3$-MeOH (7：3)

Appropriate amount of sample and reference solutions were applied with microcapillary, put the thin layer plate in an ammonia cylinder for 5 minutes, and then developed it by above solvent. Observe the spots under UV and sprayed with dragendorff reagent.

5. 5 Identified by spectral data (see them in the Chinese version).

6. Notice

6. 1 Before extract, it is important to add small amount of acetic acid to make the full expansion of medicinal herbs. It can avoid the powder expansion in percolation tube and make the extract solution difficult to flow out.

6. 2 Put two-tier moist gauze in the tube hole before poured the powder into percolation tube, then, poured the powder evenly in it and covered a layer of filter paper above it.

6. 3 Open the pistons, plus extraction solvent, then, shut down the pistons for 10 minutes to make the powder fully soaked, and then extract.

6. 4 The weight of sodium chloride is 10% of the solution volume.

7. Quetions

7. 1 What method can also be used to extract the alkaloid from *Daemonorops margaritae*? Please design the extraction processes.

7. 2 When chloride palmatine turned into tetrahydropalmatine by hydrogenation, the color changed from yellow to colorless, why?

7. 3 What methods can be used to avoid alkaloids tailing in the silica gel plate?

实验七　粉防己碱的提取、分离和鉴定

一、简介

　　粉防己（或称汉防己）是防己科千金藤属植物倒地拱（*Stephania tetrandra* S. Moore）的干燥根，主治风湿性关节疼痛，有效成分为生物碱，主要为粉防己碱（tetrandrine，又称粉防己甲素或汉防己碱）和防己诺林碱（fangchinoline，又称去甲粉防己碱或粉防己乙素），二者均属双苄基四氢异喹啉类生物碱。此外，粉防己中还含有轮环藤酚碱（cyclanoline）属原小檗碱型，是水溶性季铵生物碱。

扫码"学一学"

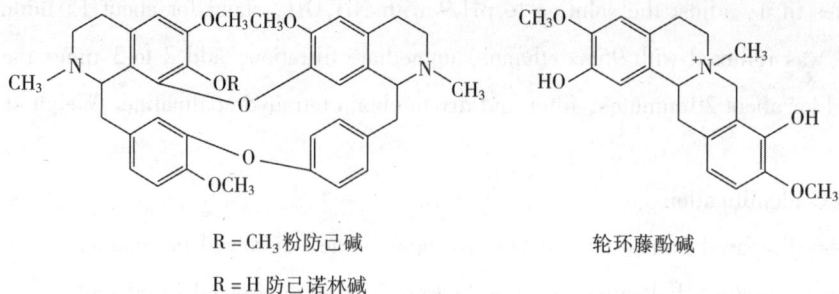

R＝CH₃ 粉防己碱

R＝H 防己诺林碱

轮环藤酚碱

二、目的

1. 了解总生物碱的提取方法。

2. 掌握酚性生物碱与非酚性生物碱的分离方法，以及水溶性生物碱的分离方法。

3. 熟悉生物碱的鉴别反应。

三、原理

粉防己碱的两个氮原子均为叔胺状态，亲脂性较强，可溶于冷苯中。防己诺林碱是粉防己碱的 O-去甲衍生物，由于酚羟基受到邻位取代基的空间位阻，以及分子内氢键的形成，使酚羟基的酸性大大减弱，因此防己诺林碱不能溶于强碱溶液。同时，酚羟基的存在使亲脂性减弱，难溶于冷苯中，借此可与粉防己碱分离。

四、仪器与试剂

1. **仪器**　圆底烧瓶（500 ml），三角瓶（500 ml），分液漏斗（500 ml），布氏漏斗，抽滤瓶，旋转蒸发仪。

2. **试剂**　粉防己粗粉，95％乙醇，1％盐酸，1％氢氧化钠，浓氨水，三氯甲烷，丙酮，苯，色谱用氧化铝，碘化汞钾试剂，碘化铋钾试剂，雷氏铵盐试剂，苦味酸试剂。

五、操作

1. **总生物碱的提取**　称取粉防己粗粉 30g，置于 250ml 圆底烧瓶中，加 95％乙醇约 80 ml，水浴加热回流 1 h，过滤，药渣再以 95％乙醇 75 ml 同法提取一次，过滤，并将瓶内药渣倒在布氏漏斗上抽干。合并两次提取液，放冷后如有絮状物析出，再抽滤一次，回收乙醇，浓缩，得总生物浸膏。

2. **亲脂性生物碱和亲水性生物碱的分离**　将总生物碱浸膏移至三角瓶中，逐渐加入 1％盐酸稀释，充分搅拌使生物碱溶解，不溶物呈树脂状析出沉淀。在水液未加足前，树脂状物常混悬于水中，继续加稀盐酸搅拌，直至加酸水时溶液不再发生混浊为止（约需 50 ml），静置，倾出上清液，瓶底的树脂状杂物以 1％盐酸少量分次洗涤，直至洗液对生物碱沉淀剂反应微弱时为止。

合并洗液与滤液，静置片刻，抽滤得澄清液体，置 500 ml 三角瓶中，滴加浓氨水调至 pH 9~10 左右，移至 500 ml 分液漏斗，加三氯甲烷 50 ml 振摇提取，分取三氯甲烷层，氨碱性水溶液再以新鲜三氯甲烷萃取数次，每次用三氯甲烷 50 ml，直至三氯甲烷抽提液的生物碱反应微弱时为止（检查时取少量三氯甲烷抽提液置表面皿上，待溶剂挥干，残留物中加稀盐酸数滴使溶解，再加生物碱沉淀剂试之），合并三氯甲烷液，此三氯甲烷液中含亲脂性叔胺碱，而三氯甲烷萃取过的氨碱性水溶液含亲水性生物碱。后者取出少量，加盐酸酸化至 pH4～5，滴加雷氏铵盐饱和水溶液，观察有无沉淀生成。

3. 亲脂性生物碱中酚性与非酚性碱的分离 三氯甲烷液移至 500 ml 的分液漏斗中，以 1％氢氧化钠水溶液 50 ml 萃取 3 次，碱水为总酚性亲脂生物碱；三氯甲烷液再用水 10 ml 各洗涤两次。三氯甲烷层加无水碳酸钾脱水干燥，过滤，将三氯甲烷全部蒸去，挥去残留溶剂后，得总非酚性亲脂生物碱。

4. 叔胺生物碱的纯化 在盛有非酚性生物碱的圆底烧瓶中，加苯 20 ml，在水浴上加热回流使生物碱溶解，倾出上清液，再用苯热提数次，合并苯溶液，如不澄清再过滤一次。回收苯，残留物加丙酮加热溶解，过滤，用热丙酮洗涤滤纸，合并滤液和洗液，置三角烧瓶中，回收丙酮至适量，放冷，加塞静置待结晶析出。析出完后用布氏漏斗抽滤，即得粉防己碱和防己诺林碱的混合物。

5. 粉防己碱和防己诺林碱的分离

（1）方法一（苯冷浸法） 取上述结晶状混合物称重，置于 50 ml 三角烧瓶中，加 5 倍量的苯冷浸，时时振摇，冷浸 1 h 后，过滤分开苯溶液和苯不溶物。苯溶液回收苯至尽，残留物以丙酮重结晶，得细针状结晶，为粉防己碱。苯不溶物待挥去残余苯后，也用丙酮重结晶，得粒状结晶，为防己诺林碱。

（2）方法二（氧化铝色谱法） 取上述结晶状混合物，以 50 倍量中性氧化铝（160 目，Ⅱ～Ⅲ级），三氯甲烷湿法装柱，将混合碱加少量三氯甲烷溶解，加于柱顶，用三氯甲烷洗脱。流分用氧化铝薄层色谱检查，丙酮－苯（1∶1）为展开剂，改良碘化铋钾为显色剂，合并相同流分，分别回收溶剂，用丙酮重结晶，即得粉防己碱和防己诺林碱。

六、生物碱的鉴定方法

1. 沉淀反应

（1）碘化汞钾试验 取样品的稀酸水溶液 1 ml，加碘化汞钾试剂（Mayer 试剂）1～2 滴，出现白色或类白色沉淀示有生物碱存在。

（2）碘化铋钾试验 取样品的稀酸水溶液 1 ml，加碘化铋钾试剂（Dragendorff 试剂）1～2 滴，出现棕红至橘红色沉淀说明有生物碱存在。

（3）雷氏铵盐试验 取样品的酸水溶液（pH4～5）1 ml，加雷氏铵盐试剂数滴，出现沉淀说明有生物碱存在。

（4）苦味酸试验 取样品的中性水溶液，加苦味酸的饱和水溶液，生成黄色沉淀说明有生物碱存在。

2. 薄层色谱

（1）吸附剂 硅胶 CMC－Na 色谱板。

（2）样品 ①粉防己碱；②防己诺林碱；③总生物碱；均溶于乙醇中。

（3）展开剂 ①三氯甲烷－乙醇（10∶1，或10∶0.7），氨气饱和；②甲苯－丙酮－甲醇（4∶5∶1），氨气饱和；③三氯甲烷－丙酮－甲醇（4∶5∶1），氨气饱和。

（4）显色剂 碘化铋钾。

3. 光谱法鉴别

（1）粉防己碱 无色针晶，熔点 217～218 ℃，不溶于水、石油醚，易溶于乙醇、甲醇、丙酮、三氯甲烷、苯和烯酸水溶液。

UV(λ_{max}, nm): 282.5, 257

IR(ν_{max}, KBr, cm^{-1}): 2920, 2825, 1540, 1568, 1490, 1250, 1220, 1090, 830, 813

MS(m/z): 622, 621, 515, 485, 448, 396, 395, 381, 364, 349, 198, 175, 174

^{1}H-NMR(δ): 3.92, 3.74, 3.37, 3.18 (12H, 4×OCH$_3$), 2.62, 2.33 (6H, 2×N-CH$_3$), 7.43-6.00 (10H, m, Ar-H)

^{13}C-NMR(δ): 61.4 (C-1), 44.1 (C-3), 22.1 (C-4), 128.0 (C-4α), 105.8 (C-5), 151.2 (C-6), 137.9 (C-7), 148.2 (C-8), 133.0 (C-8α), 134.9 (C-9), 116.2 (C-10), 146.9 (C-11), 149.3 (C-12), 111.6 (C-13), 122.6 (C-14), 41.9 (C-α), 63.9 (C-1′), 42.6 (C-3′), 25.3 (C-4′), 128.1 (C-4′α), 112.7 (C-5′), 148.5 (C-6′), 143.7 (C-7′), 120.0 (C-8′), 127.8 (C-8′α), 134.9 (C-9′), 132.4 (C-10′), 121.7 (C-11′), 153.6 (C-12′), 121.7 (C-13′), 129.9 (C-14′), 38.3 (C-α), 42.3 (N-CH$_3$), 42.6 (N′-CH$_3$)

（2）防己诺林碱　六面体结晶（丙酮），熔点 134～136 ℃；溶解性能与粉防己碱相似，但在苯中的溶解度小于粉防己碱，在乙醇中的溶解度大于粉防己碱。

UV（λ_{max}, nm）: 282, 259

IR（ν_{max}, KBr, cm^{-1}）: 3420, 1610, 1580, 1510, 1460, 1380, 1320, 1260, 1060, 1120

MS(m/z): 608, 607, 471, 417, 382, 381, 367, 350, 335, 321, 192, 174

^{1}H-NMR(δ): 3.92, 3.74, 3.33 (9H, 3×OCH$_3$), 2.58, 2.33 (6H, 2×N-CH$_3$), 7.50-6.03 (10H, m, Ar-H)

^{13}C-NMR(δ): 61.2 (C-1), 44.0 (C-3), 21.8 (C-4), 122.8 (C-4α), 104.7 (C-5), 145.7 (C-6), 134.5 (C-7), 141.8 (C-8), 132.2 (C-8α), 134.7 (C-9), 115.9 (C-10), 143.4 (C-11), 146.7 (C-12), 111.2 (C-13), 122.5 (C-14), 37.9 (C-α), 63.5 (C-1′), 44.0 (C-3′), 25.0 (C-4′), 127.5 (C-4′α), 112.0 (C-5′), 148.4 (C-6′), 149.0 (C-7′), 128.1 (C-8′α), 134.8 (C-9′), 132.2 (C-10′), 121.6 (C-11′), 153.4 (C-12′), 121.6 (C-13′), 129.5 (C-14′), 41.7 (C-α), 42.1 (N-CH$_3$), 42.2 (N′-CH$_3$).

七、思考题

1. 粉防己甲素和粉防己乙素在结构上有哪些共同点和不同点？这些异、同点在理化性质上有哪些反映？实验过程中，我们如何利用他们的共性和个性？

2. 如何利用薄层色谱条件判断分离得到了什么化合物及其纯度？

3. 分离水溶性与脂溶性生物碱的常用方法有哪些？

Experiment Ⅷ　Extraction, Isolation and Identification of Alkaloids in "Fen Fang Ji"

1. Introduction

"Fen Fang Ji"（also called "Han Fang Ji"）is the dried root of *Stephania tetrandra* S. Moore, and used to treat the ache of rheumatoid arthritis. Alkaloid components are considered as the active ingredients in "Fen Fang Ji" mainly composed of tetrandrine and fangchinoline, both of which are bisbenzyl tetrahydroisoquinoline alkaloids containing two diphenyl ether linkages. Cyclan-

扫码"练一练"

66

oline is a water-soluble quaternary ammonium base having protoberberine skeleton.

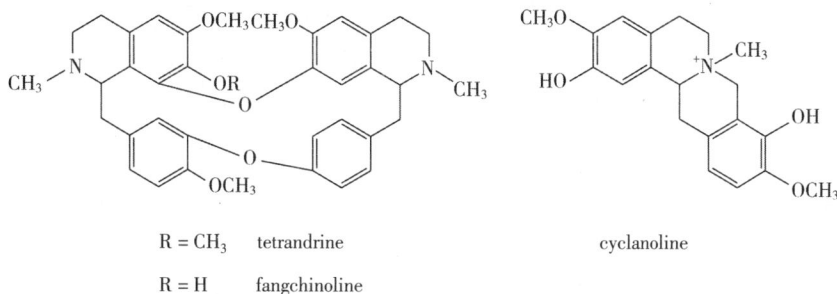

R = CH₃　　tetrandrine

R = H　　　fangchinoline

cyclanoline

2. Purposes

2. 1 Learn how to extract the total alkaloids from raw material.

2. 2 Master the isolation method of phenolic, non-phenolic, and water-soluble alkaloids from total alkaloids.

2. 3 Be familiar with the identification reactions of alkaloids.

3. Principles

Tetrandrine shows a strong lipophilicity because both nitrogen atoms are in the state of tertiary amine, so it can be dissolved in benzene. Fangchinoline is the O-demethyl derivation of tetrandrine, the acidity of whose phenolic hydroxyl is weakened by the effect of adjacent steric hindrance and the presence of intramolecular hydrogen bond, so it can't be dissolve in strong basic solution. However, the phenolic hydroxyl group can reduce the lipophilicity. As a result, fangchinoline is difficult to be dissolved in benzene, so we can separate these two alkaloids in this way.

4. Apparatus and reagents

4. 1 Apparatus

Round-bottom flask (250 ml), conical flask (500 ml), separationg funnel (500 ml), büchner funnel, suction filtering funnel, rotary evaporator.

4. 2 Reagents

Crude powder of the roots of *Stephania tetrandra*, 95 % EtOH, 1 % HCl, 1 % NaOH, concertrated ammonia liquor, CHCl₃, acetone, benzene, toluene, MeOH, anhydrous potassium carbonate, alumina, Mayer reagent, Dragendorff reagent, Ammonium reineckate reagent, Hager reagent.

5. Procedures

5. 1 Extraction of the total alkaloids

To weigh the crude powder of the roots of *Stephania terandra* about 30 g in a 250 ml round-bottom flask, add 200 ml 95 % ethanol and reflux for 1 hours on water bath. Then filter and extract the residue again in the same way by 150 ml 95% ethanol. Filter and pour the residue onto a Buchner funnel in order to extrude the solution. Combine the extractions, cool, filter once more if there are floccules appeared. Evaporate the ethanol and a thick residue obtained, which is the total alkaloids part.

5. 2 The isolation of the lipophilic and the hydrophilic alkaloids

Transfer the total alkaloids to a conical flask, add 1% hydrochloric acid slowly, stir thoroughly to make alkaloids fully dissolved, insolubles deposit as resin-like. Add 1% hydrochloric acid continually while stirring until no more insolubles yield (about 100 ml used), remain undisturbed, and pour the upper solution. Wash the resin-like left in bottle by 1% hydrochloric acid for several times up to the time that the washes show weak reaction to the precipitant agent of alkaloids.

Combine the washes and filtrate, keep still for a moment, filter to get clear liquid. Transfer to a 500 ml conical flask, drip concentrated ammonia liquor till pH 9, then transfer to 500 ml separating funnel. Add chloroform 50 ml, shake, collect the chloroform layer, the alkaline water keep on extracting with chloroform for several times until the chloroform layer show weak reaction to the precipitant agent of alkaloids. Combine the chloroform solution, which contains the lipophilic tertiary amine alkaloid. The hydrophilic alkaloids were left in the ammoniacal liquor, acidify a little by hydrochloric acid to pH 4 ~ 5, drop saturate solution of ammonium reineckate, observe the appearance of deposition.

5. 3 The separation of phenolic and non-phenolic lipophilic alkaloids

Transfer the chloroform solution to a 500 ml separating funnel, extract with 1% sodium hydroxide solution 50 ml three times, then elute with 10 ml water two times, collect the chloroform layer. Dry the solution by anhydrous potassium carbonate, filter. When the solvent was evaporated, the total non-phenolic alkaloids resulted.

5. 4 Purify of tertiary amine alkaloid

Add benzene 20 ml to a round-bottom flask containing non-phenolic alkaloids, reflux on the water bath to make alkaloids dissolve, pour out the upper solution, repeat several times, combine the benzene solution, filter if necessary. Evaporate the solvent, the residue dissolved in acetone warmly, filter, wash the filter by warm acetone, and combine the filtrate and washes. Transfer the solution to a conical flask, concentrate the acetone to small volume, cool, seal, keep standing and wait for the crystal secreting out. Collecte the crystals with a suction on a Büchner funnel, the mixture of tetrandrine and fangchinoline is obtained.

5. 5 The isolation of tetrandrine and fangchinoline

Method I : Percolating by benzene

Transfer the mixture mentioned above into a 50 ml conical flask, percolate with five times of benzene for an hour and shake at intervals, filter with a suction on a Büchner funnel to separate the benzene solution and materials undissolved in benzene. Remove the solvent of the benzene solution, recrystallize the residue by acetone, tetrandrine is obtained as fine needle crystal. After the solvent volatilization, the materials undissolved in benzene are recrystallized by acetone also, fangchinoline is obtained as granular crystal.

Method II : Alumina column chromatography

The mixture mentioned above is purified by alumina column chromatography with chloroform as the eluent. The column is loaded by wet packing method, and the mixture add to the top of the column after dissolved in a little of chloroform. The fractions are identified by alumina TLC, with acetone-benzene（1∶1）as developing agent and Dragendorff agent as chromogenic reagent. Combine the same fraction, evaporate the solvent respectively, recrystallize the residue by acetone, tetrandrine and fangchinoline are obtained.

6. General Identification for Alkaloids

6.1 Precipitation reaction

Mayer reagent test　Add Mayer reagent 1~2 drops to 1ml dilute acidic solution of sample. The white-like depositions appearance displays the occurrence of alkaloids.

Dragendorff reagent test　Add Dragendorff reagent 1~2 drops to 1ml dilute acidic solution of sample. It shows the occurrence of alkaloids that saffron to nacarat depositions appearance.

Ammonium reineckate reagent test　Add Ammonium reineckate reagent several drops to 1ml acidic solution of sample（pH4~5）. It shows the occurrence of alkaloids that depositions appearance.

Hager reagent test　Add saturated Picric acid reagent 1~2 drops to neutral solution of sample. It shows the occurrence of alkaloids that yellow depositions appearance.

6.2 Thin-layer chromatography

Adsorbent：silica gel CMC-Na plate for TLC.

Sample：① tetrandrine，② fangchinoline，③ total alkaloids；All of these samples dissolved in ethanol.

Developing Solvent：① $CHCl_3$ – EtOH（10∶1, or 10∶0.7）, saturated with NH_3

② toluene-acetone-MeOH（4∶5∶1）, saturated with NH_3

③ $CHCl_3$-acetone-MeOH（4∶5∶1）, saturated with NH_3

Chromogenic reagent：Dagendorff reagent.

6.3 Identified by spectral data

Tetrandrine, colorless needles, m. p. 217~218℃, Insoluble in water, petroleum ether. Dissolves in ethanol, methanol, acetone, chloroform, benzene, and dilute acid.

（See them in Chinses version）

7. Questions

1. What are the common and different characteristics of the structures between tetrandrine and fangchinoline? What are their exhibitions on physical and chemical property? How to make use of them in the course of experiment?

2. How to identify the isolated compounds and estimate their purity by TLC?

3. What are the general methods of the isolation between the lipophilic and the hydrophilic alkaloids?

实验八　大黄中游离蒽醌的提取、分离和鉴定

一、简介

大黄为蓼科植物掌叶大黄 *R. heum palmatum* L.、唐古特大黄 *R. tanguticum* Maxim. ex

扫码"学一学"

Balf. 或药用大黄 *R. officinale* Baill. 的干燥根及根茎。味苦，性寒。具有泻热通肠，凉血解毒，逐瘀通经的功效。其主要成分为蒽醌衍生物，总量约 3% ~ 5%，部分游离，大部分以苷的形式存在。其中大黄酸、大黄素和芦荟大黄素具有抗菌、抗感染作用，大黄酚具有止血作用，大黄粗提物、大黄素和大黄酸具有抗肿瘤作用，番泻苷类具有泻下作用，鞣酸类化合物具有止泻作用。

二、目的

1. 掌握蒽醌苷元的提取方法——两相水解法。
2. 掌握 pH 梯度萃取法分离酸性成分的原理及操作技术。
3. 掌握硅胶柱色谱法分离的原理和操作技术。
4. 掌握羟基蒽醌类化合物的鉴定方法。
5. 掌握蒽醌类化合物乙酰化和甲基化的原理和方法。

三、原理

大黄中蒽醌类化合物以结合态和游离态两种形式存在，主要化合物如下。

大黄酸（rhein）为黄色针状结晶，熔点 321 ~ 322℃，330℃分解。能溶于碱、吡啶，微溶于乙醇、苯、三氯甲烷、乙醚和石油醚，不溶于水。

大黄素（emodin）为橙黄色针状结晶（乙醇或冰醋酸），熔点 256 ~ 257℃，能升华。易溶于乙醇、碱液，微溶于乙醚、三氯甲烷，不溶于水。

芦荟大黄素（aloe-emodin）为橙色针状结晶（甲苯），熔点 223 ~ 224℃。易溶于热乙醇，可溶于乙醚、苯、碳酸钠和氢氧化钠水溶液。

大黄酚（chrysophanol）为橙黄色六方形或单斜形结晶（乙醇或苯），熔点 196 ~ 197℃，能升华。易溶于沸乙醇，可溶于甲醇、乙醇、丙酮、三氯甲烷、苯、乙醚和氢氧化钠水溶液，微溶于石油醚、冷乙醇，不溶于水、碳酸钠和碳酸氢钠水溶液。

大黄素甲醚（physcion）为砖红色单斜针状结晶，熔点 203 ~ 207℃（苯），溶于苯、三氯甲烷、吡啶及甲苯，微溶于乙酸及乙酸乙酯，不溶于甲醇、乙醇、乙醚和丙酮。

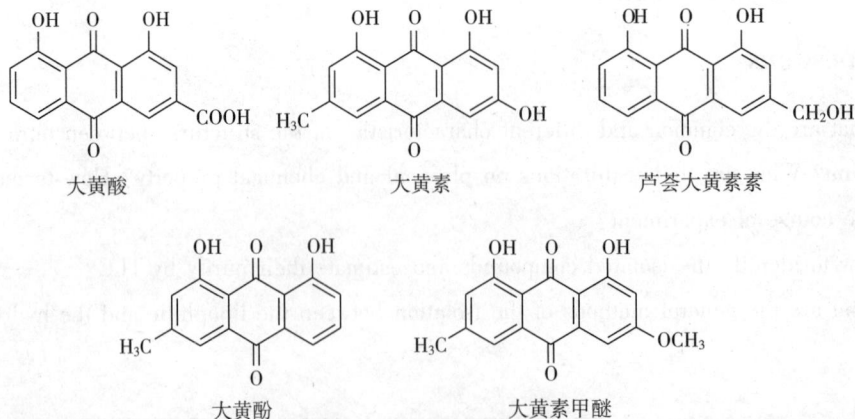

大黄酸　　　　　　　　大黄素　　　　　　　芦荟大黄素素

大黄酚　　　　　　　大黄素甲醚

羟基蒽醌苷类：大黄素甲醚葡萄糖苷（physion monoglucoside），黄色针状结晶，熔点 235℃；芦荟大黄素葡萄糖苷（aloe-emodin monoglucoside），熔点 239℃；大黄素葡萄糖苷（emodin monoglucoside），浅黄色针状结晶，熔点 190 ~ 191℃；大黄酸葡萄糖苷（rhein 8-monoglucoside），熔点 266 ~ 267℃；大黄酚葡萄糖苷（chrysophanol monoglucoside），熔点

245~246℃。

因大黄中蒽醌存在形式以结合状态为主，为提高游离蒽醌的得率，采取酸水解和乙醚萃取相结合的方法即两相水解法进行提取。

依据 5 种苷元酸性强弱不同，采用 pH 梯度萃取法分离。苷元酸性强弱顺序为：大黄酸 > 大黄素 > 芦荟大黄素 > 大黄素甲醚 > 大黄酚。

依据 5 种苷元极性不同，采用硅胶柱色谱法分离。苷元极性强弱顺序为：大黄酸 > 芦荟大黄素 > 大黄素 > 大黄素甲醚 > 大黄酚。

四、仪器与试剂

1. **仪器**　水浴，圆底烧瓶（250 ml，50 ml），冷凝管，烧杯（100ml，250 ml），抽滤瓶（500 ml），分液漏斗（500 ml），旋转蒸发仪，循环水泵，紫外灯，展开缸，点样毛细管，锥形瓶（250 ml），锥形瓶（50 ml，15 个）。

2. **试剂**　10% 硫酸，乙醚，2.5% NaHCO₃，2.5% Na₂CO₃，5% Na₂CO₃，0.5% NaOH，滤纸（5 cm×8 cm），薄层硅胶 G，0.8% CMC - Na，浓盐酸，冰醋酸，丙酮，乙酸乙酯，氢氧化钾，硫酸二甲酯，三氯甲烷，无水硫酸钠，无水碳酸钾，无水吡啶，乙酸酐，乙醇，醋酸镁。

五、展开剂及对照品

1. **展开剂**　PE - EtOAc - HOAc（6∶4∶0.2 或 20∶3∶0.6）。
2. **对照品**　大黄酸，大黄素，芦荟大黄素，大黄酚，大黄素甲醚。

六、操作

1. **酸水解及总蒽醌苷元的提取**　取大黄 10 g，粉碎，加 10% 硫酸水溶液 50 ml 充分搅拌湿润后装入 250 ml 圆底烧瓶中，加乙醚 50 ml 热水浴上回流提取 1 h，过滤得滤液，药渣继续用乙醚 50 ml 回流提取 1 h，过滤，合并 2 次乙醚提取液（t）于 500 ml 的分液漏斗中，加 100 ml 蒸馏水洗至中性备用。

2. **蒽醌苷元类成分的分离**

【方法一：pH 梯度萃取法】

（1）大黄酸的分离和精制　将上述乙醚提取液（t），用 2.5% 碳酸氢钠水溶液 120ml 分 3 次萃取，每次 40 ml，充分振摇，静置至彻底分层，分出碱水层置 250ml 的烧杯中（注意观察萃取时溶液的颜色变化）。碱水层小心滴加浓盐酸至 pH 3（注意：不断搅拌，并观察酸化时溶液的颜色变化），放置沉淀，待沉淀析出完全后过滤，沉淀用水洗至近中性，干燥，称重，即为大黄酸粗品。沉淀干燥后，样品加冰醋酸 10ml 加热溶解，趁热过滤，滤液放置析晶，过滤，用少量冰醋酸淋洗结晶，得黄色针晶为大黄酸。

（2）大黄素的分离和精制　上述经 2.5% 碳酸氢钠萃取过的乙醚液（a），用 2.5% 碳酸钠水溶液 120ml 萃取 3 次，每次 40 ml，充分振摇，静置至彻底分层，分出碱水层置 250ml 的烧杯中。碱水层小心滴加浓盐酸至 pH 3（注意事项：同上），放置沉淀，待沉淀析出完全后，过滤，沉淀用水洗至近中性，干燥，称重，即为中等酸性部分，主要含大黄素。用 15ml 丙酮热溶，趁热过滤，滤液静置，析出橙色针晶，过滤后，用少量丙酮淋洗结晶，得大黄素。

扫码"看一看"

（3）芦荟大黄素的分离和精制　　上述经 2.5% 碳酸钠萃取过的乙醚液（b），用 5% 碳酸钠水溶液 120ml 萃取 3 次，每次 40 ml，分出碱水层置 250ml 的烧杯中，调至 pH 3，放置沉淀，过滤，沉淀用水洗至近中性，干燥，称重，用 10ml 乙酸乙酯精制，得黄色针晶芦荟大黄素。

（4）大黄酚和大黄素甲醚的分离　　上述除去芦荟大黄素后余下的乙醚层（c），用 0.5% 氢氧化钠水溶液 90 ml 萃取 3 次，每次 30 ml，合并氢氧化钠萃取液于 250 ml 的烧杯中，调至 pH 3，析出黄色沉淀，过滤，水洗至中性，干燥，称重，即为弱酸性部分，主要含大黄酚和大黄素甲醚。余下乙醚液（d）水洗至中性，蒸馏回收乙醚。

（5）薄层板　　硅胶 G 薄层色谱板。

①展开剂：PE－EtOAc－HAc（6∶4∶0.2 或 20∶3∶0.6）。

②样品：乙醚液（t，a－d）。

【方法二：硅胶柱色谱法】

（1）装柱

1）方法一　　干法装柱。取 100～200 目柱色谱用硅胶粉 15 g，用小漏斗倒入 2 mm×300 mm 柱底部垫有少许精制棉且下端活塞打开的色谱柱内，轻轻敲打色谱柱，使柱内硅胶粉均匀充实，得干硅胶色谱柱。

2）方法二　　湿法装柱。取 100～200 目柱色谱用硅胶粉 15g 于 100 ml 的烧杯中，加入石油醚搅拌均匀至无气泡，倒入 20 mm×300 mm 柱底部垫有少许精制棉且下端活塞打开的色谱柱内，轻轻敲打色谱柱，流 3 个柱体积石油醚，使柱内硅胶粉均匀充实，得湿硅胶色谱柱。

（2）上样　　取上述提取的总羟基蒽醌苷元乙醚液于 250 ml 圆底烧瓶中，浓缩至干，用少量乙醚转移至蒸发皿中，加柱色谱用硅胶粉 1 g，搅拌于通风橱中晾干，得均匀样品粉末，仔细加入硅胶色谱柱的上端，轻敲色谱柱使样品粉末平整，上加约 0.5 cm 厚的保护硅胶。

（3）洗脱与收集　　首先，用石油醚－丙酮（9∶1）或石油醚－乙酸乙酯（7∶3）混合溶剂洗脱，使用 250 ml 锥形瓶收集洗脱液。柱上黄色色带开始流出时，更换 50 ml 锥形瓶，10～15 ml 为一流分，顺序编号。直至三个黄色色带流出，改用石油醚－丙酮（5∶5）混合溶剂或乙酸乙酯洗脱至橙色色带流出为止。每个流分经薄层色谱检查，相同斑点者合并，分别回收溶剂，浓缩放置析晶。

3. 大黄素的三甲基化和三乙酰化

（1）三甲基化

1）方法一　　将 1.68 g（30 mmol）氢氧化钾溶于 3 ml 蒸馏水中，加入大黄素 2.7 g（10 mmol），搅拌下慢慢滴加硫酸二甲酯 3.78 g（30 mmol），混合物回流反应 2 h。反应液用三氯甲烷（50 ml×3）萃取，无水硫酸钠干燥得粗产品，硅胶柱色谱分离纯化［流动相为石油醚－丙酮（3∶1）］，三氯甲烷重结晶得黄色晶体，干燥，称重，计算收率，测定熔点。

2）方法二　　向圆底烧瓶中分别加入 0.8 g（3 mmol）大黄素、120 ml 丙酮、12g 无水碳酸钾，不断搅拌下滴加 8ml 硫酸二甲酯。混合物加热回流 24h，反应液浓缩至原体积的一半，加蒸馏水 50ml 稀释，过滤收集黄色沉淀。母液蒸除大部分丙酮又可以得到一部分产物，合并粗产物，三氯甲烷重结晶，得大黄素三甲基化衍生物，称重，计算收率，测定熔点。

（2）三乙酰化 取大黄素 200 mg，置于 50 ml 干燥的圆底烧瓶中，加 4 ml 无水吡啶溶解，再加 5ml 乙酸酐摇匀，水浴上加热回流 30 min，放冷，将反应液在搅拌下倾入 100 ml 冰水中，一直搅拌至油滴消失，固体沉淀析出，抽滤，滤饼用水洗涤，干燥后用 95% 的乙醇重结晶，得粉末状结晶。

4. 鉴定

（1）化学鉴定

①碱液试验 分别取上述分离所得游离蒽醌类化合物结晶各少许于小试管中，加 95% 乙醇 1ml 溶解，再加 10% 氢氧化钠水溶液 2~3 滴，观察溶液颜色变化。

②醋酸镁试验 分别取上述分离所得游离蒽醌类化合物结晶各少许于小试管中，加 95% 乙醇 1ml 溶解，再加 0.5% 醋酸镁乙醇液 2~3 滴，观察溶液颜色变化。

（2）薄层色谱鉴定

吸附剂：硅胶 G - CMC - Na 板，于 110 ℃烘半小时。

样品溶液：自制大黄酸、大黄素、芦荟大黄素、大黄酚和大黄素甲醚少量，以适量乙醇溶解。

对照品溶液：大黄酸、大黄素、芦荟大黄素、大黄酚和大黄素甲醚对照品适量，以适量乙醇溶解。

展开剂：Pet - EtOAc - HAc（6∶4∶0.2 或 20∶3∶0.6）。

用毛细管各吸取样品和对照品溶液适量，点于同一硅胶 G 薄层板上，用上述展开剂展开。薄层板吹干后，在日光和紫外光灯（365nm）下观察色斑，再置于浓氨气中熏或喷 5% 醋酸镁乙醇溶液，在日光下检视，斑点变成红色。

（3）光谱法鉴别 大黄中 5 种游离蒽醌类化合物的光谱数据如下。

1）大黄酚

UV（λ_{max}^{MeOH}, nm）：225.2，255.2，270.2，287.2，429.0

IR（ν_{max}，KBr，cm^{-1}）：3050，1672（C = C），1601，1563，901，868，839

EI-MS（m/z）：254（M$^+$，100），239（M-CH$_3$），237（M-OH），226（M-CO），198（M-2CO）.

^{1}H-NMR（CDCl$_3$，500MHz）δ：7.04（2-H，1H，brs），7.58（4-H，1H，brs），7.77（5-H，1H，d，J = 7.5Hz），7.63（6-H，1H，t，J = 8.22Hz），7.26（7-H，1H，t，J = 8.6Hz），2.44（CH$_3$，3H，s），12.06（OH，1H，s），11.94（OH，1H，s）

^{13}C-NMR（CDCl$_3$，125MHz）δ：162.4（C-1），124.5（C-2），149.3（C-3），121.3（C-4），119.9（C-5），136.9（C-6），124.3（C-7），162.6（C-8），192.4（C-9），181.8（C-10），133.2（C-4α），115.8（C-8α），113.6（C-9α），133.5（C-10α），22.3（CH$_3$）

2）大黄素甲醚

UV（λ_{max}^{MeOH}, nm）：220.0，253.0，263.8，292.0，433.0

IR（ν_{max}，KBr，cm^{-1}）：3430，1670，1625，1564，970，873

EI-MS（m/z）：284（M$^+$），256（M-CO），269（M-CH$_3$）

^{1}H-NMR（CDCl$_3$，500 MHz）δ：7.07（2-H，1H，brs），7.62（4-H，1H，d，J = 1.3Hz），7.36（5-H，1H，d，J = 2.5Hz），6.68（7-H，1H，d，J = 2.5Hz），2.45（CH$_3$，3H，s），3.94（OCH$_3$，3H，s），12.31（OH，1H，s），12.11（OH，1H，s）

^{13}C-NMR（CDCl$_3$，125MHz）δ：165.2（C-1），124.5（C-2），148.5（C-3），121.3（C-4），110.3（C-5），162.5（C-6），107.8（C-7），166.5（C-8），190.8（C-9），182.0（C-10），133.2（C-4α），108.2（C-8α），113.7（C-9α），135.2（C-10α），22.2（CH$_3$），56.1（OCH$_3$）

3）大黄素

UV（λ_{max}^{MeOH}，nm）：220.8，252.2，264.8，288.0，440.1

IR（ν_{max}，KBr，cm^{-1}）：3378，1620，1475，1439，1366，1329，874，759

EI-MS（m/z）：270（M$^+$，100），255（M-CH$_3$），253（M-OH），242（M-CO），214（M-2CO），213（M-H-2CO）

^{1}H-NMR（DMSO-d_6，500 MHz）δ：7.04（2-H，1H，d，J=2.3Hz），7.37（4-H，1H，brs），7.05（5-H，1H，brs），6.52（7-H，1H，d，J=2.3Hz），2.36（CH$_3$，3H，brs），12.00（1H，s，α-OH），11.92（1H，s，α-OH），11.32（1H，s，β-OH）

^{13}C-NMR（DMSO-ds，125MHz）δ：164.5（C-1），107.8（C-2），165.6（C-3），108.8（C-4），120.4（C-5），148.2（C-6），124.0（C-7），161.5（C-8），189.7（C-9），181.1（C-10），135.0（C-4α），（C-8α），108.8（C-9α），132.7（C-10α），113.2（C-4），21.4（CH$_3$）

4）芦荟大黄素

UV（λ_{max}^{MeOH}，nm）：222（3.99），254（2.05），277（sh），287（1.26），430（0.89）

IR（ν_{max}，KBr，cm^{-1}）：3353（OH），1720，1670，1622，1568，1471，1448

EI-MS（m/z）：270［M$^+$］，242［M-CO］，225［M-CO-OH］，214［M-2CO］

^{1}H-NMR（DMSO-d_6，500MHz）δ：7.23（2-H，1H，d，J=1.2Hz），7.63（4-H，1H，d，J=1.2Hz），7.76（5-H，1H，dd，J=2.0，8.0Hz），7.64（6-H，1H，dd，J=8.0，8.0Hz），7.34（7-H，1H，dd，J=2.0，8.0Hz），11.92（1H，s，C$_1$-OH），11.85（1H，s，C$_8$-OH），5.59（1H，-CH$_2$OH），4.60（2H，s，-CH$_2$OH）

^{13}C-NMR（DMSO-d_6，125MHz）：161.5（C-1），119.3（C-2），153.7（C-3），117.1（C-4），120.6（C-5），137.3（C-6），124.4（C-7），161.3（C-8），191.6（C-9），181.3（C-10），133.0（C-4α），114.3（C-8α），115.8（C-9α），133.2（C-10α），62.0（CH$_2$OH）

5）大黄酸

UV（λ_{max}^{MeOH}，nm）：203（1.88），226（1.99），258（1.21），287（287），433（0.52）

IR（ν_{max}，KBr，cm^{-1}）：3407（—OH），1707（—COOH），1673，1624，1560，1449

FAB-MS m/z（%）：285［M+1］$^+$，257［M+1-CO］，241［M+1-COOH］

^{1}H-NMR（DMSO-d_6，500MHz）δ：7.39（2-H，1H，d，J=3.0Hz），8.18（4-H，1H，d，J=3.0Hz），7.85（5-H，1H，dd，J=2.6，7.3Hz），7.76（6-H，1H，dd，J=7.3，7.9Hz），7.47（7-H，1H，dd，J=2.6，7.9Hz），11.87（1H，s，br），11.87（1H，s，br）

^{13}C-NMR（DMSO-d_6，125MHz）δ：161.6（C-1），125.1（C-2），138.1（C-3），119.3（C-4），1119.9（C-5），138.1（C-6），124.9（C-7），161.9（C-8），192.0（C-9），181.6（C-10），134.4（C-4a），119.9（C-8α），116.7（C-9α），133.8（C-10α），165.9（COOH）

七、注意事项

1. 水解液酸性强，避免用手直接接触。

2. 分液漏斗使用前需进行检漏。

3. 柱色谱时玻璃器皿干燥，无水；装柱时，下端活塞应打开；洗脱剂不能低于柱平面。

4. 在大黄素三甲基化中，硫酸二甲酯和氢氧化钾的用量是关键，当其用量与大黄素的摩尔比为 1 : 1 时，主要产物为大黄素 6 位甲基化衍生物，而摩尔比为 3 : 1 时，大黄素三甲基化衍生物为主要产物。

5. 由于本实验所制大黄素不能满足本部分实验需要，若实验室开展大黄素三甲基化或三乙酰化实验，需提前购买大黄素。

6. 利用本实验教材中的方法，大黄中五个游离蒽醌类成分均可以被分离，各学校可以根据各自实验室的条件和学时调节实验内容，例如多数学校只以分离大黄素为目标。

八、思考题

1. 试述大黄中 5 种游离羟基蒽醌类化合物的酸性和极性顺序，并说明理由。
2. 试述 pH 梯度萃取法的原理，并说明适用于哪些中药成分的分离。
3. 试述湿法装柱和干法装柱各有什么优缺点？

扫码"练一练"

Experiment Ⅷ Extraction, Isolation and Identification of Free Anthraquinones in Rhei Radix et Rhizoma

1. Introductions

Radix et Rhizoma Rhei (Dahuang) is the dried root and rhizome of *R. heum palmatum* L. , *R. tanguticum* Maxim. ex Balf and *R. officinale* Baill. in Polygonaceae family. Bitter-tasted and cold-natured. It has effects of clearing away heat, purging fire, removing toxins, promoting blood circulation to remove blood stasis, and dispelling heat from the blood to stop bleeding.

The main constituents in Radix et Rhizoma Rhei are anthraquinone derivatives (3% ~5%), some are free and most are glycosides. The antibacterial, anti-infective active ingredients are rhein, emodin and aloe-emodin. The main haemostati ingredient is chrysophanol. The crude extracts of Dahuang, emodin and rhein have inhibitive effect towards experimental tumor. The main lapactic ingredients are sennosides. Besides, Dahuang also contains10% -30% tannic compounds, which has antidiarrheal effect.

2. Purposes

2. 1 Learn the extraction method ofanthraquinone aglycones-two-phase hydrolysis.

2. 2 Learn theprinciple and operation of separating acidic constituents with pH gradient extraction method.

2. 3 Learn theprinciple and operation of isolation using silica gel column chromatography (silica gel CC).

2. 4 Learn theidentification method of hydroxyl-anthraquinones compounds.

2. 5 Learn theprinciple and method of acetylation and methylation of anthraquinone compounds.

3. Principles

Theanthraquinones in Dahuang exists in bound and free states. The main compounds are as follows.

Rhein are yellow needle crystals, m. p. 321 ~ 322℃, decomposition point 330℃. Rhein dissolves in alkali aqueous solution and pyridine. It's slightly soluble in ethanol, benzene, chloroform, ethyl ether and petroleum ether, practically insoluble in water.

Emodin are orange yellow needle crystals (ethanol or glacial acetic acid), m. p. 256 ~ 257℃, which can be sublimated. It's easily soluble in ethanol and aqueous alkali, slightly soluble in ethyl ether and chloroform, insoluble in water.

Aloe-emodin are orange needle crystals (methylbenzene), m. p. 223 ~ 224℃. It's easily soluble in warm ethanol, soluble in ethyl ether, benzene, sodium carbonate and sodium hydroxide aqueous solution.

Chrysophanol are orange yellow six square ormonoclinic crystals (ethanol or benzene), m. p. 196 ~ 197℃, and can be sublimated. It's easily soluble in boiling ethanol, soluble in methanol, ethanol, acetone, chloroform, benzene, ethyl ether and sodium hydroxide aq, slightly soluble in petroleum ether and cold ethanol, insoluble in water, sodium carbonate and Sodium Hydroxide aq.

Physcion are brick redmonoclinic needle crystals, m. p. 203 ~ 207℃ (benzene). It's soluble in benzene, chloroform, pyridine, and methylbenzene, slightly soluble in acetic acid and acetic ether, insoluble in methanol, ethanol, ethyl ether and acetone.

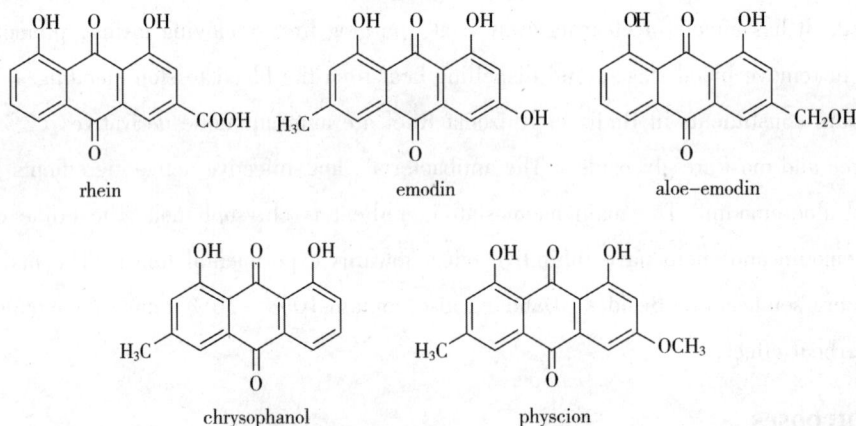

rhein   emodin   aloe-emodin

chrysophanol   physcion

Hydroxyanthraquinone glycosides: physion monoglucosides are yellow needle crystals, m. p. 235℃; aloe-emodin monoglucoside, m. p. 239℃; emodin monoglucoside, pale yellow needle crystals, m. p. 190 ~ 191℃; rhein 8-monoglucoside, m. p. 266 ~ 267℃; chrysophanol monoglucoside, m. p. 245 ~ 246℃, etc.

Anthroquinones in Dahuang mainly exist in bound form. In order to obtain more free anthraquinones, the method of combining acid hydrolysis and extraction with ethyl ether is used (two-phase hydrolysis).

According to different acidity offive aglycones, pH gradient extraction method is used to separate them. The sequence of aglycone acidity is as follows: rhein > emodin > aloe-emodin > physcion > chrysophanol.

According to different polarities of five aglycones, silica gel CC can be used to separate them. The sequence of aglycone polarities is: rhein > aloe-emodin > emodin > physcion > chrysophanol.

4. Apparatus and reagents

4.1 Apparatus

Thermostat-controlled water bath, round bottomed flask (250 ml, 50 ml), condenser, beaker (100 ml, 250 ml), suction flask (500 ml), separating funnel (500 ml), rotary evaporation, circulating pump, vacuum pump, UV-lamp, developing chamber for TLC, microcapillary, conical flask (250 ml), conical flask (50 ml, 15 pieces).

4.2 Reagents

10% H_2SO_4, ethyl ether, 2.5% $NaHCO_3$, 2.5% Na_2CO_3, 0.5% $NaOH$, filter paper, (5 cm ×8 cm) silica gel G for TLC, 0.8% CMC-Na, HCl, glacial acetic acid, acetone, ethyl acetate, KOH, dimethyl sulphate, $CHCl_3$, anhydrous sodium sulfate, anhydrous potassium carbonate, anhydrous pyridine, acetic anhydride, ethanol.

5. Developing solvents and references

5.1 Developing Solvents

PE-EtOAc-HOAc (6 : 4 : 0.2 or 20 : 3 : 0.6)

5.2 References

Rhein, emodin, aloe-emodin, chrysophanol, physcion.

6. Procedures

6.1 Acid Hydrolysis and Extraction of Total Anthraquinone Aglycones

In a 250 ml flask place 10g of Dahuang crude powder moistened with 50 ml of 10% aqueous H_2SO_4, and 50ml of ethyl ether refluxing on water bath for 1 hours. Then filter and extract the residue again in the same way with 50ml of ethyl ether for 1 hour. Filter and combine the filtrate to 500 ml separating funnel. Wash them with 100ml of distilled water to neutral, and separate the ethyl ether extract (t), which is total hydroxyanthraquinone aglycones.

6.2 Isolation

6.2.1 pH Gradient extraction

6.2.1.1 The isolation and purification of rhein　Extract the above ethyl ether extract (t) with 120ml of 2.5% aqueous $NaHCO_3$ for three times (40ml each time), shake and layer thoroughly, separate the aqueous alkali layer into a 250 ml beaker. Add concentrated HCl carefully under stirring to pH 3 (observing the color change while extraction and acidification), keep the solution until educes thoroughly, filter it to get the precipitation, wash the precipitation with water to near neutral, dry and weigh it, which is the strong acidity part, mainly rhein. After the precipitation is dried, add 10ml of glacial acetic acid and make it dissolved as more as possible by warming on a water bath. Filter the hot solution to remove insoluble impurities, allow the solution cool. The yellow needle crystals appear gradually. Filter them and wash with glacial acetic acid, then obtain rhein.

6. 2. 1. 2 The isolation and purification of emodin　Extract the above ethyl ether extract (a) having been extracted by aqueous NaHCO₃ with 120ml of 2.5% aqueous Na₂CO₃ for three times (40ml each time), shake and layer thoroughly, separate the aqueous alkali layer into a 250 ml beaker. Add concentrated HCl carefully under stirring to pH 3 (observing the color change while extraction and acidification), keep the solution until educes thoroughly, filter it to get the precipitation, wash the precipitation with water to near neutral, dry and weigh it, which is the moderate acidity part, mainly emodin. After the precipitation is dried, add 15ml of acetone and make it dissolved as more as possible by warming on a water bath. Filter the hot solution to remove insoluble impurities, allow the solution cool. The yellow needle crystals appear gradually. Filter them and wash with acetone, then obtain emodin.

6. 2. 1. 3 The isolation and purification of aloe-emodin　Extract the above ethyl ether extract (b) having been extracted by aqueous 2.5% Na₂CO₃ with 120ml of 5% aqueous Na₂CO₃ for three times (40ml each time), separate the aqueous alkali layer into a 250 ml beaker. Add concentrated HCl carefully under stirring to pH 3, keep the solution until educes thoroughly, filter it to get the precipitation, wash the precipitation with water to near neutral, dry and weigh it, recrystallize it with 10 ml of acetic ether, then obtain aloe-emodin.

6. 2. 1. 4 The isolation and purification of chrysophanol and physcion　Extract the above ethyl ether extract (c) having been extracted by aqueous 5% Na₂CO₃ with 90ml of 0.5% aqueous NaOH for three times (30 ml each time), separate the aqueous alkali layer into a 250 ml beaker. Add concentrated HCl carefully under stirring to pH 3, keep the solution until educes thoroughly, filter it to get the precipitation, wash the precipitation with water to near neutral, dry and weigh it, which is the weak acidity part, mainly chrysophanol and physcion. Wash the surplus ethyl ether solution (d) to neutrality, distill it to recover ethyl ether.

6. 2. 1. 5 The TLC tracking check　Silica gel G-CMC-Na.

Developing Solvents：PE-EtOAc-HAc (6：4：0.2 or 20：3：0.6)

Sample：ethyl ether solution (t, a-d)

6. 2. 2 Silica gel CC

6. 2. 2. 1 Packing the column

Method Ⅰ: Dry packing. Fill a few purified cotton at the bottom of 20mm × 300mm chromatographic column (CC), puts a small funnel above it and open the inferior piston. Pour 15g of 100 ~ 200 mesh silica gel powder into the CC and tap softly to make the silica gel powder filled uniformly, then obtain the dry silica gel CC.

Method Ⅱ: Wet packing. In a 100ml beaker mix 15g of 100 ~ 200 mesh silica gel powder and petroleum ether uniformly without air bubble. Pour them into the 20mm × 300mm CC which has a few purified cotton at the bottom and the inferior piston opened. Three times petroleum ether as much as the column volume flow through the column and tap softly to make the silica gel powder filled uniformly, then obtain the wet silica gel CC.

6. 2. 2. 2 Add sample　Ethyl ether extract (t), which is total hydroxyanthraquinone aglycones. Pour the above ethyl ether solution containing total hydroxyanthraquinone aglycone into 250ml

flask, condense them to dry. Transfer them to evaporating basin with a few ethyl ether, add 1g silica gel powder, stir and dry them in fuming cupboard, obtain the sample powder. Then add them at top of CC carefully, tap softly to make the sample powder smooth, add silica gel powder about 0.5cm thickness to protect the plane.

6.2.3 Elution and collection

At first, elute with PE-Me$_2$CO (9∶1) or PE-EtOAc (7∶3), collect the eluent with 250ml conical flask. Change 50ml conical flask while the yellow color strip begins to be eluted, every fraction contains 10 ~ 15ml numbered sequencely, until the three yellow color strips are eluted. Then elute with PE-Me$_2$CO (5∶5) or EtOAc until orange color strip flows out. Every fraction is analyzed with TLC, combine the identical spots, recover the solvent and educe the crystals respectively.

6.3 Trimethylation and triacetylation of emodin

6.3.1 Trimethylation

Method 1: Dissolve 1.68 g (30 mmol) of KOH in 3ml of distilled water, add 2.7 g (10 mmol) of emodin, and dropwise 3.78 g (30 mmol) of dimethyl sulphate slowly under stirring. The mixtures are refluxed on a water bath for 2 hours, then extracted with CHCl$_3$ (50ml × 3) and dried with anhydrous sodium sulfate. The crude products obtained are isolated and purified with silica gel CC (PE-acetone = 3∶1 as mobile phase), recrystallize it with CHCl$_3$, obtain the yellow crystals, dry and weigh them, calculate the yield and determine the melting point.

Method 2: In around-bottomed flask place 0.8g (3mmol) of emodin, 120ml acetone, 12g of anhydrous potassium carbonate, dropwise 8 ml of dimethyl sulphate under stirring. The mixtures are refluxed for 24 hours, and condensed to half, add 50 ml of distilled water. Filter and collect the yellow precipitate, obtain another products while distilling the majority acetone in mother liquor. Combine the crude product, recrystallize it with CHCl$_3$, obtain trimethylation derivate of emodin, dry and weigh them, calculate the yield and determine its melting point.

6.3.2 Triacetylation

In a 50ml round-bottomed flask place 200 mg of emodin dissolved with 4ml of anhydrous pyridine, and 5ml of acetic anhydride, refluxon a water bath for 30 minutes. Cool and pour them into 100ml of ice water, stir until the oil drops disappear and precipitation appear. Filtering with sucking filtration, the filter cake obtained are washed with water. After dried, recrysted with 95% ethanol and obtain powder crystals.

6.4 Identification

6.4.1 Chemical identification

6.4.1.1 Alkali test　Put appropriate amount of prepared free anthraquinones into the small test tube respectively, add 1ml of 95% ethanol, 2 ~ 3 drops of 10% aqueous NaOH, observe the solution color.

6.4.1.2 Magnesium Acetate test　Put appropriate amount of prepared free anthraquinones into the small test tube respectively, add 1ml of 95% ethanol, 2 ~ 3 drops of magnesium acetate ethanol solution, observe the solution color.

6.4.2 TLC

Adsorbent：Silica Gel G-CMC-Na, roasted at 110 ℃ for half an hour

Samples：Prepared Rhein, emodin, aloe-emodin, chrysophanol and physcion, dissolved in ethanol

References：Rhein, emodin, aloe-emodin, chrysophanol and physcion for reference, dissolved in ethanol

Developing solvent：PE-EtOAc-HAc (6 : 4 : 0.2 or 20 : 3 : 0.6)

Appropriate amount of sample and reference solutions were applied with microcapillary, developed by above solvent. Observe the spots either directly or exposing the sheet to UV light (365 nm) before and after the sheet was perfumed with NH_3 or sprayed with 5% magnesium acetate ethanol solution.

6.4.3 Identified by Spectral Data (See them in the Chinese part).

7. Notices

7.1 Acidity of thehydrolysis solution is strong, avoid touch directly with hands.

7.2 Examine whether the separating funnel is leak before using.

7.3 When CC, make sure glasswares dry without water. Open the inferior piston when packing. The eluant should not be lower than the plane of the column.

7.4 In the process of emodin trimethylation, the key is the amount of dimethyl sulphate and KOH. While the mole ratio of them and emodin is 1 : 1, the main product is 6-methylation emodin, and the ratio is 3 : 1, the main product is trimethylation emodin.

7.5 Please buy emodin in advance if you want to carry out trimethylation and triacetylation of emodin because prepared emodin can't satisfy the experiment.

7.6 The five free hydroxyanthraquinones in Dahuang can be isolated using the method of this experiment teaching material. Every university can adjust the experiment content according to the conditions of your lab and time e.g., the experiment object only is isolation of emodin in many universities.

8. Questions

8.1 Compare the acidity and polarity of the five free hydroxyanthraquinones in Dahuang.

8.2 What are the principles of pH gradient extraction method? What kinds of traditional Chinese medicine can be separated with the method?

8.3 What advantages and disadvantages are there wet packing column and dry packing column?

实验九　前胡中香豆素的提取、分离和鉴定

一、简介

前胡为伞形科植物白花前胡 *Peucedanum praeruptorum* Dunn 的干燥根。前胡具有散风清

热，降气化痰的功效，用于风热咳嗽痰多，痰热喘满，咳痰黄稠，是一味常用的中药。

前胡的主要活性成分为香豆素类化合物，已分离出白花前胡甲素（Praeruptorin A）、白花前胡乙素（Praeruptorin B）、白花前胡丙素（Praeruptorin C）和白花前胡丁素（Praeruptorin D）等化合物。此外，前胡中还含有挥发油、色原酮、黄酮、聚炔、木脂素、简单苯丙素衍生物等成分。现代药理研究表明：前胡中的香豆素类成分具有抗脑缺血、抗心衰及扩张血管降低血压等作用。

二、目的

1. 掌握脂溶性香豆素类化合物的提取方法。
2. 熟悉使用化学反应和 TLC 法鉴定香豆素的方法。

三、原理

白花前胡甲素、乙素、丙素和丁素等是前胡中的主要成分，其中白花前胡甲素与白花前胡丙素为一对光学异构体，白花前胡乙素与白花前胡丁素是一对光学异构体，由于这几种香豆素均以苷元的形式存在，故极性较小，可溶于石油醚中。故以石油醚为溶剂，采用索氏提取法进行提取，便可直接得到香豆素的粗晶。

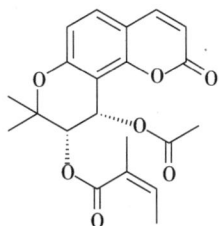

白花前胡甲素　　　　　　　　白花前胡乙素

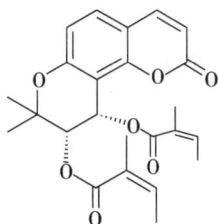

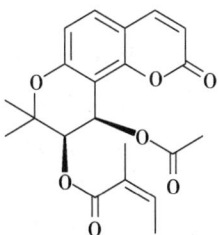

白花前胡丙素　　　　　　　　白花前胡丁素

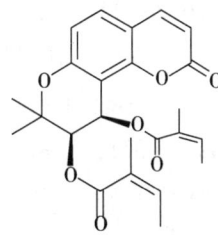

四、仪器与试剂

1. **仪器**　索氏提取器，圆底烧瓶（250ml），冷凝管，紫外灯，展开缸，点样毛细管。
2. **试剂**　石油醚（60～90℃），乙酸乙酯，氢氧化钠，盐酸，乙醇，异羟肟酸铁试剂，硅胶 GF254。

五、展开剂及对照品

1. **展开剂**　石油醚（60～90℃）–乙酸乙酯（3∶1）。
2. **对照品**　白花前胡甲素。

六、操作

1. **提取**　取白花前胡根粉末 100 g，置索氏提取器中，加石油醚（60～90℃）回流提取 3 h，提取液浓缩至 20 ml 左右，冷却，放置，有淡黄白色结晶析出。

2. **精制**　滤取提取液中析出的结晶，用石油醚反复洗结晶，得到 1g 左右的前胡总香豆素的粗晶。

3. **香豆素的检识**

（1）显色反应　取样品少许溶于乙醇中，加异羟肟酸铁试剂观察颜色。

（2）开闭环反应　取样品少许加稀氢氧化钠溶液 1～2 ml，加热，观察现象；再加稀酸试液几滴，观察所产生现象。

（3）荧光　取样品少许溶于三氯甲烷中，用毛细管点于滤纸上，于紫外灯下观察荧光。

（4）香豆素的薄层鉴定

样品溶液：取上述得到的香豆素粗晶少量，溶于三氯甲烷中。

对照品溶液：白花前胡甲素对照品溶于三氯甲烷中。

吸附剂：硅胶 GF_{254} 薄层板。

展开剂：石油醚（60～90℃）－乙酸乙酯（3∶1）

用毛细管吸取样品和对照品溶液适量，点于薄层板上，用上述展开剂展开。晾干后，在紫外灯（254nm）下检视。

（5）光谱法鉴别

1）白花前胡甲素

UV 258nm，357nm

IR（ν_{max}^{KBr}, cm^{-1}）3422（羟基），1658（羰基），1602，1502（苯基）

^{1}H-NMR（CDCl$_3$）δ：6.24（1H，d，J = 9.6 Hz，H-3），7.61（1H，d，J = 9.6 Hz，H-4），7.36（1H，d，J = 8.6 Hz，H-5），6.81（1H，d，J = 8.6 Hz，H-6），5.40（1H，d，J = 5.0 Hz，H-3′），6.55（1H，d，J = 5.0 Hz，H-4′），1.44（3H，s，2′-CH$_3$），1.48（3H，s，2′-CH$_3$），6.14（1H，br. q，J = 7.2 Hz，H-3″），1.96（3H，br. d，J = 7.2 Hz，H-4″），1.87（3H，br. s，5″-CH$_3$），2.11（3H，s，2‴-CH$_3$）

^{13}C-NMR（CDCl$_3$）δ：159.9（C-2），113.1（C-3），143.3（C-4），129.1（C-5），114.3（C-6），156.6（C-7），106.9（C-8），153.9（C-9），112.4（C-10），77.6（C-2′），69.7（C-3′），60.9（C-4′），22.9（2′-CH$_3$），24.9（2′-CH$_3$），166.4（C-1″），126.8（C-2″），139.8（C-3″），15.7（C-4″），20.4（C-5″），169.9（C-1‴），20.6（C-2‴）

EI-MS（m/z）386（M$^+$）

2）白花前胡乙素

IR（ν_{max}^{KBr}, cm^{-1}）3600－2800（羟基），1640（羰基），1600，1500（苯基）

^{1}H-NMR（CDCl$_3$）δ：6.21（1H，d，J = 9.6 Hz，H-3），7.58（1H，d，J = 9.6 Hz，H-4），7.35（1H，d，J = 8.6 Hz，H-5），6.80（1H，d，J = 8.6 Hz，H-6），5.44（1H，d，J = 5.0 Hz，H-3′），6.69（1H，d，J = 5.0 Hz，H-4′），1.45（3H，s，2′-CH$_3$），1.48（3H，s，2′-CH$_3$），6.11（1H，br. q，J = 7.2 Hz，H-3″），1.98（3H，d，J = 7.2 Hz，H-4″），1.84（3H，br. s，5″-CH$_3$），6.02（1H，br. q，J = 6.8 Hz，3‴-H），1.95（3H，d，J = 6.8 Hz，4‴-CH$_3$），1.82（3H，br. s，5‴-

CH_3)

^{13}C-NMR（CDCl$_3$）δ:159. 7（C-2），113. 2（C-3），143. 1（C-4），129. 1（C-5），114. 3（C-6），156. 6（C-7），107. 4（C-8），154. 3（C-9），112. 4（C-10），77. 4（C-2′），70. 1（C-3′），60. 9（C-4′），22. 4（2′-CH$_3$），25. 3（2′-CH$_3$），166. 4（C-1″），127. 3（C-2″），139. 8（C-3″），15. 7（C-4″），20. 4（C-5″），166. 2（C-1‴），127. 0（C-2‴），138. 4（C-3‴），15. 5（C-4‴），20. 3（C-5‴）

EI-MS（m/z）426（M$^+$）

七、思考题

1. 香豆素类化合物的提取还可以采用哪些方法？

2. 根据白花前胡甲素、乙素、丙素和丁素的结构特点，设计实验方案对它们的混合物进行分离。

扫码"练一练"

Experiment Ⅸ　Extraction，Isolution and Identification of Coumarins from Peucedani Radix

1. Introduction

Peucedani radix（Qianhu）is the dried root of *Peucedanum praeruptorum* Dunn. It has the effect of clearing away wind and heat，lowering adverse-rising energy and dissipating phlegm，often used for cough and excessive phlegm due to wind-heat evil，dyspneal fullness，yellow and thick expectoration. It is a commonly used traditional chinese medicine.

The main constituents in Qianhu are coumarins，Praeruptorin A，Praeruptorin B，Praeruptorin C and Praeruptorin D，etc have been isolated. In addition，Qianhu also contains volatile oils，chromones，flavonoids，polyalkynes，lignans and simple phenylpropanoids derivatives，etc. Modern pharmacological researches show that coumarins in Qianhu have the effects of anti-cerebral ischemia，anti-congestive heart failure and lowering blood pressure by distending blood vessel.

2. Purposes

2. 1 Learn the extraction method of lipophillic coumarins.

2. 2 Familiar with the identification methods of coumarins by chemical reaction and TLC.

3. Principles

Praeruptorin A，Praeruptorin B，Praeruptorin C and Praeruptorin D are the main constituents of Qianhu. Praeruptorin A and Praeruptorin C are optical isomers，while Praeruptorin B and Praeruptorin D are optical isomers. In Qianhu，all coumarins above are aglycones with low polarity and can be dissolved in petroleum ether，so they can be extracted by soxhlet's with petroleum ether as solvent.

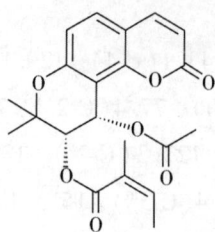

Praeruptorin A

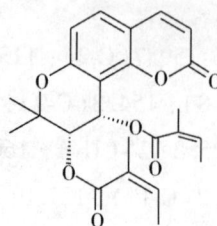

Praeruptorin B

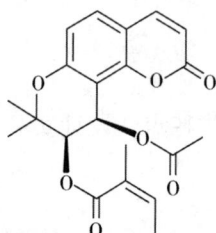

Praeruptorin C

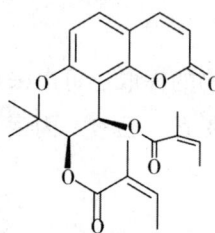

Praeruptorin D

4. Apparatus and reagents

4.1 Apparatus

Soxhlet's, round bottomed flask (250ml), condenser, UV-lamp, developing chamber for TLC, macrocapillary (1mm).

4.2 Reagents

Petroleum ether (60 ~ 90℃), EtOAc, NaOH, HCl, ethanol, Ferric hydroxamic acid reagents, silica gel GF254.

5. Developing solvents and references

5.1 Developing solvents

Petroleum ether (60 ~ 90℃)-EtOAC (3 : 1)

5.2 References

Praeruptorin A

6. Procedures

6.1 Extraction

In a Soxhlet's place 100g of Qianhu powders, extract with petroleum ether (60 ~ 90℃) for 3 hours, then condense the extract to 20 ml, cool it to room temperature, stand for to get yellowish white crystals.

6.2 Purification

Filter the above extract to get crystals, wash them with petroleum ether repeatedly to get 1g of crude crystals of total coumarins.

6.3 Identification

6.3.1 Color reaction

Dissolve the samples with ethanol, add Ferric hydroxamic acid reagents, and observe the phenomena.

6.3.2 Open and closed ring reaction

In a test tube place a little sample, add 1~2ml of NaOH solution, heat, observe the phenomena; Then add some drops of dilute HCl, observe the change of phenomena.

6.3.3 Fluorescence

Dissolve the little sample in chloroform, spot it on the filter paper with microcapillary, observe the fluorescence with UV lamp.

6.3.4 TLC of coumarins

Samples：Prepared crude crystals, dissolved in chloroform.

References：Praeruptorin A for reference, dissolved in chloroform.

Adsorption：silica gel GF_{254}.

Developing Solvent：Petroleum ether (60~90℃) – EtOAC (3∶1)

Appropriate amount of sample and reference solutions are applied with microcapillary, developed by solvents above. Observe the spots by exposing the sheet to UV light (254nm).

6.3.5 Identified by spectral data (See them in Chinese part.)

7. Questions

7.1 What are the other methods to extract coumarins?

7.2 Accoridng to the structure characteristics of Praeruptorin A, Praeruptorin B, Praeruptorin C and Praeruptorin D, design a procedure to separate them.

实验十　何首乌二苯乙烯苷的提取、分离和鉴定

一、简介

二苯乙烯苷属多羟基芪类化合物（polyhydrostilbenes），广泛存在于藓类和高等植物中，天然的二苯乙烯苷主要以二苯乙烯苷元侧链结合一个单糖基的形式存在。何首乌中二苯乙烯苷是其降血脂及抑制动脉粥样硬化的主要有效成分。

何首乌为蓼科蓼属植物何首乌 *Polygonum multiflorum* Thunb. 的干燥块根，是历版《中国药典》收载品种。现代药理研究证明，何首乌具有抗衰老、增强机体免疫功能、降血脂、抗微生物、通便等多种作用。2, 3, 5, 4′ – 四羟基二苯乙烯 – 2 – O – β – D – 葡萄糖苷是何首乌二苯乙烯苷类成分中的主要化合物，为何首乌特有的有效成分。目前，以何首乌二苯乙烯总苷为原料研制开发的治疗动脉粥样硬化的新药已进入临床试验阶段。

二、目的

1. 掌握二苯乙烯苷类化合物的提取分离方法。
2. 掌握二苯乙烯苷类成分的理化性质。
3. 掌握硅胶柱色谱的使用方法。

三、原理

2, 3, 5, 4′ – 四羟基二苯乙烯 – 2 – O – β – D – 葡萄糖苷（是天然存在的二苯乙烯苷），

扫码"学一学"

分子式为 $C_{20}H_{22}O_9$，分子量为 406.39，为白色无定形粉末，熔点为 184~186℃，易溶于水、甲醇、乙醇，难溶于亲脂性有机溶剂。因此提取时，一般采用水、稀乙醇等溶剂进行提取。二苯乙烯类化合物的纯化通常采用各种柱色谱方法进行纯化，常用的色谱方法有硅胶柱色谱法、大孔吸附树脂色谱法、高效液相色谱法等。本实验中采用了常用的硅胶柱色谱方法进行纯化，以获得纯品。

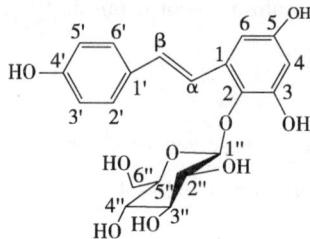

2，3，5，4′－四羟基二苯乙烯－2－O－β－D－葡萄糖苷
（2，3，5，4′－stilbene glucoside）的化学结构

四、仪器与试剂

1. **仪器** 圆底烧瓶（500 ml），三角烧瓶（500 ml×2，50 ml×3），玻璃漏斗（10 cm×2.5 cm），布氏漏斗＋抽滤瓶（50 ml），乳钵，玻璃色谱柱（2.5 cm×50 cm），滴管（3只），试管（20 ml×30 支），蒸发皿，量筒（500 ml，50 ml 各1支），分液漏斗（1000 ml），加液球（500 ml）。超声仪，旋转蒸发仪，两孔水浴锅，循环水泵，电吹风，铁架台＋铁夹＋铁圈（2套），紫外灯，展开缸，点样毛细管（1mm），脱脂棉，玻璃棒。

2. **试剂** 甲醇，正丁醇，乙醇，柱色谱用硅胶（200~300 目），浓硫酸，硅胶 GF254板，滤纸，碘。

五、展开剂及对照品

1. **展开剂** 二氯甲烷：乙酸乙酯：甲醇：乙酸：水＝18：3：8：2：2
2. **对照品** 2，3，5，4′－四羟基二苯乙烯－2－O－β－D－葡萄糖苷

六、操作

1. 二苯乙烯苷的提取和纯化

（1）提取 取何首乌药材粉末（过40目筛）50g，置500ml 圆底烧瓶中，加蒸馏水400ml，超声提取2h。取出圆底烧瓶，滤纸常压过滤，药渣用100 ml 水洗，收集滤液。滤液（约500ml）置分液漏斗中，用正丁醇萃取（200ml）×5 次，合并萃取液，减压回收至干，得总二苯乙烯苷。

（2）柱色谱 取总二苯乙烯苷0.5g，置蒸发皿中，用5ml 甲醇溶解，加约2g硅胶拌样，烘干。称取柱色谱用硅胶25g，以干法装入玻璃色谱柱中。拌样硅胶同法装柱。最后加入少量硅胶覆盖。以乙酸乙酯：甲醇（15：1）混合溶剂200ml 进行洗脱，流速为1~1.5 ml/min。洗脱液用20ml 试管分管接收。收集的洗脱液以对照品对照进行薄层检测，合并含目标成分的洗脱液，回收溶剂至干，得2，3，5，4′－四羟基二苯乙烯－2－O－β－D－葡萄糖苷粗品。

（3）重结晶　取约 300mg 2，3，5，4′－四羟基二苯乙烯－2－O－β－D－葡萄糖苷 6~10 ml，乙酸乙酯溶解，抽滤，收集滤液。滤液边搅拌边加入 3~4 ml 三氯甲烷至析出沉淀，静置 10 min，析晶。抽滤，用三氯甲烷少许洗涤结晶，得 2，3，5，4′－四羟基二苯乙烯－2－O－β－D－葡萄糖苷精制品。干燥，称重，计算得率。如不纯，可重复一次重结晶操作。

2. 二苯乙烯苷的鉴别　2，3，5，4′－四羟基二苯乙烯－2－O－β－D－葡萄糖苷稀乙醇溶液，滴于滤纸上，再滴加稀乙醇扩散后，紫外光灯下显持久的亮蓝色荧光；蒽醌衍生物则出现黄色至浅棕色环，紫外光灯下呈棕色至棕红色荧光。

3. 二苯乙烯苷的硅胶薄层色谱鉴定

薄层板：硅胶 GF254 板。

样品溶液：自制 2，3，5，4′－四羟基二苯乙烯－2－O－β－D－葡萄糖苷少量，以适量乙醇溶解。

对照品溶液：2，3，5，4′－四羟基二苯乙烯－2－O－β－D－葡萄糖苷标准品乙醇溶液。

展开剂：二氯甲烷：乙酸乙酯：甲醇：乙酸：水（18：3：8：2：2）。

用毛细管各吸取样品和对照品溶液适量，点于硅胶板上，用上述展开剂展开。硅胶板吹干后，在可见光及紫外灯下观察色斑；用碘熏硅胶板后在可见光下观察色斑变化；碘挥发后，均匀喷以 15% 硫酸乙醇液，电吹风加热，斑点显红色→灰褐色的变化。

4. 二苯乙烯苷的 HPLC 色谱鉴定

色谱条件：色谱柱为 TOSOH　TSK gel OSD－100V 柱（4.6 mm×250 mm，5 μm）。

流动相：乙腈：水（25：75）。

检测波长：320 nm。

流速：1.0 ml/min。

柱温：25 ℃。

二苯乙烯苷对照品约 2 mg，精密称定，置于 10ml 量瓶中，50% 乙醇溶解定容，得浓度为 200 μg/ml 的对照品溶液。自制二苯乙烯苷样品 2mg 同法制备样品溶液。对照品及样品溶液过 0.45 μm 微孔滤膜，吸取 10 μl 滤液，注入高效液相色谱柱，采用上述色谱条件，记录色谱图。对照品及样品均在 7.882 min 处在现色谱峰（图 2－1）。

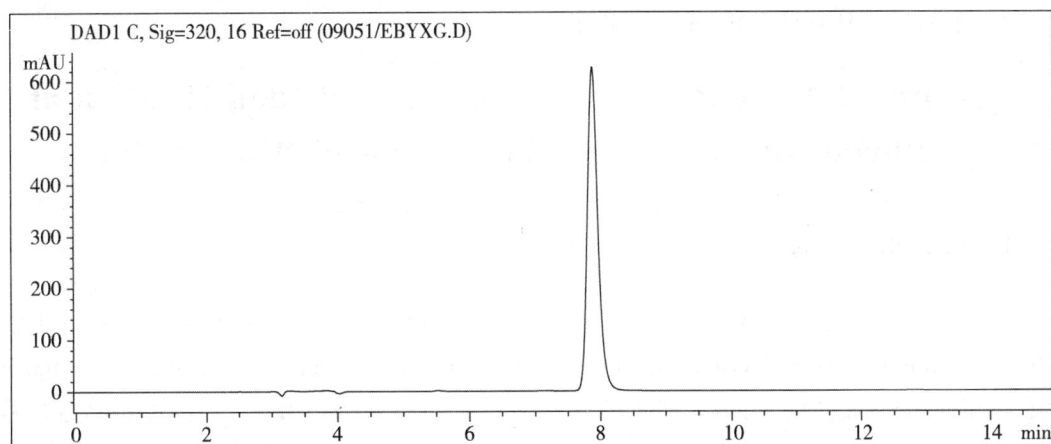

图 2－1　二苯乙烯苷对照品 HPLC 色谱图

5. 光谱法鉴定

UV (λ_{max}, nm): 214, 321

IR (ν_{max}, KBr): 3405 (broad, OH); 1605, 1559, 1541, 1514 (⬡—); 1245, 1194 (C—O—C)

EI-MS (m/z): 244 (100%, M-glc), 228, 197, 169, 144, 107, 94, 60

ESI-MS (m/z): 407.1 [M+H]$^+$, 429.2 [M+Na]$^+$; 405.1 [M−H]$^-$, 811.2 [2M−H]$^-$

^{1}H-NMR (600 MHz, DMSO-d_6)δ: 7.66 (1H, d, $J=16.8$ Hz, H-α), 7.43 (2H, d, $J=8.4$ Hz, H-2′, 6′), 6.87 (1H, d, $J=16.8$ Hz, H-β), 6.73 (2H, d, $J=8.4$ Hz, H-3′, 5′), 6.52 (1H, d, $J=3.0$ Hz, H-6), 6.16 (1H, d, $J=3.0$ Hz, H-4), 4.39 (1H, d, $J=7.8$ Hz, H-1″)

^{13}C-NMR (150 MHz, DMSO-d_6)δ: 157.1 (C-4′), 154.6 (C-5), 150.6 (C-3), 136.3 (C-2), 131.9 (C-1), 128.5 (C-1′), 128.4 (C-β), 128.1 (C-2′, 6′), 120.5 (C-α), 115.4 (C-3′, 5′), 106.6 (C-1″), 102.6 (C-4), 101.0 (C-6), 77.1 (C-5″), 76.0 (C-3″), 73.9 (C-2″), 69.3 (C-4″), 60.7 (C-6″)

七、注意事项

1. 本实验用药材以生首乌为佳，制首乌中二苯乙烯苷含量较低。

2. 样品进行硅胶拌样时可使用水浴锅加热的方法挥干溶剂，但要注意温度不能过高（60 ℃以下）。同时，还应边加热边搅拌，以免造成样品受热不均崩样，损失样品。

3. 进行柱色谱时，洗脱剂流速不宜过快，洗脱液的流速一般以 30 ~ 60 min 内流出液体的毫升数与所用吸附剂的重量（克）相等为合适。

4. 进行硅胶柱色谱时，一般从第 2 管开始就有目标物被洗脱下来，实验时应注意采用二苯乙烯苷的鉴别方法监测。

八、思考题

1. 二苯乙烯苷和蒽醌类化合物在理化性质上有哪些不同之处？如何鉴别？

2. 简述硅胶吸附色谱的原理及其应用。

扫码"练一练"

Experiment Ⅹ Extraction, Isolation and Identification of Stilbene Glucoside from Polygoni Multiflori Radix

1. Introductions

Stilbene glucosides, a kind of polyhydrostilbene, distribute in moss and higher plants widely. While the natural stilbene glucosides are often in existence in the form of a monosaccharide linked with stilbene aglycon. The stilbene glucosides from Polygoni Multiflori Radix (Heshouwu) are the main effective compounds with antilipidic anti-atherosclerotic activity.

Dried root of *Polygonum multiflorum* Thunb, well known as Heshouwu, is one of the most popular traditional medicinal herbs in China, and is officially listed in the Chinese Pharmacopoeia. It

has been reported to possess many effects, such as antilipidic, antioxidation, antibacteria, lubricating intestine and detoxification and so on. 2, 3, 5, 4′-stilbene glucoside, the most abundant in the total stilbene glucosides of Heshouwu, is the characteristic active compound of it. Now, the new anti- atherosclerotic drug, made from the total stilbene glucosides of Heshouwu, has been entered the clinical trial phase.

2. Purposes

2.1 Learn the extraction, isolation method of stilbene glucosides.

2.2 Familiar with the main properties of stilbene glucosides.

2.3 Learn the utilization of silica gel column chromatography.

3. Principles

2, 3, 5, 4′-stilbene glucoside are white amorphous powder. Its molecular formula is $C_{20}H_{22}O_9$, and the molecular weight is 406.39, m. p. 184~186℃. 2, 3, 5, 4′-stilbene glucoside is soluble in water, methanol, and ethanol, but insoluble in common organic solvents. So it can be extracted with water and ethanol, and purified by various column chromatography, such as HPLC, macroporous adsorption resin, and silica gel column chromatography. Here, silica gel column chromatography was applied to obtain purified 2, 3, 5, 4′-stilbene glucoside.

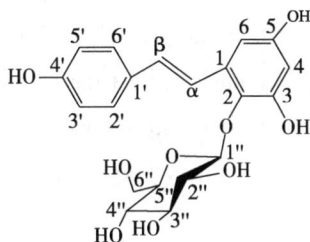

2, 3, 5, 4′-stilbene glucoside

4. Apparatus and reagents

4.1 Apparatus

Round bottom flasks (500 ml), conical flask (500 ml×2, 50ml×5), glass funnel (10 cm×2, 5cm), Büchner's filter + suction flask (500 ml), mortar, glass chromatographic column (2.5×50 cm), droppers, tubes (20 ml×30), evaporating basin, graduated flask (500ml, 50ml), separatory funnel (1000 ml), feeding ball (500 ml), ultrasonic apparatus, rotary evaporator, thermostat-controlled water-bath, vacuum pump, electric hair-drier, iron stand + iron clip + iron ring, UV-lamp, developing chamber for TLC, glass sample capillary tube (1mm), cotton wool, glass rod.

4.2 Reagents

Methanol, n-butanol, ethanol, silica gel (200~300 mesh), concentrated sulfuric acid, TLC plate (GF254), filter paper, iodine.

5. Developing solvents and references

5. 1 Developing Solvents

CH_2Cl_2 : EtOAc : MeOH : AcOH : H_2O (18 : 3 : 8 : 2 : 2)

5. 2 References

2, 3, 5, 4'-stilbene glucoside

6. Procedures

6. 1 Isolation and purification of 2, 3, 5, 4'-stilbene glucoside

6. 1. 1 Isolation

In a 500ml round bottom flask place 50g powder of Heshouwu, and 400ml of distilled water. Extract with ultrasonic wave for 2h, then filter to collect filtrate, wash the gruffness with 100ml water. Place the 500ml filtrate in a 1000ml separatory funnel, extract with 200ml *n*-BuOH for 5 times, combine *n*-BuOH extraction, remove *n*-BuOH by rotary evaporator under reduced pressure to get crude total stilbene glucosides.

6. 1. 2 Silica gel column chromatography

In an evaporating basin place 0. 5g of crude total stilbene glucosides, add 2g silica gel to absorb the sample, evaporate the solvent on a water bath (not exceeding 60℃). Mount 2. 5 × 50cm chromatography column with 25g silica gel dry powder, load sample with the same method, cover the sample with a thin layer of silica gel. Elute with about 200ml mixed solvent of EtOAc : MeOH (15 : 1) with the flow rate of 1 ~ 1. 5 ml/min. Collect the elution with tubes (20ml/tube), respectively. Examine the elution by TLC contrasted with reference, combine the same elution containing the objective compound, remove solvent by rotary evaporator under reduced pressure to obtain crude 2, 3, 5, 4'-stilbene glucoside.

6. 1. 3 Recrystallization

Dissolve 300 mg of crude 2, 3, 5, 4'-stilbene glucoside in about 6 ~ 10 ml of ethyl acetate, make 2, 3, 5, 4'-stilbene glucoside dissolved as more as possible by warming on a water bath. Filter the hot solution to remove insoluble impurity. To the filtrate add 3 ~ 4ml chloroform while stirring the mixture to precipitation, stand for 10min then precipitate crystals of 2, 3, 5, 4'-stilbene glucoside. Filter the mixed solution to get purified 2, 3, 5, 4'-stilbene glucoside. Weigh and calculate the yield.

6. 2 Examination of stilbene glucoside

Drop 2, 3, 5, 4'-stilbene glucoside ethanol solution on filter paper, scatter with diluted alcohol. Observe filter paper under UV light, show permanent sapphirine flurescence, while anthraquinone derivatives brown to brownish red fluorescence.

6. 3 Identification of 2, 3, 5, 4'-stilbene glucoside by TLC Chromatography

TLC plate: Silica gel GF254 plate.

Sample: Prepared 2, 3, 5, 4'-stilbene glucoside, dissolved in ethanol.

Reference: 2, 3, 5, 4'-stilbene glucoside for reference, dissolved in ethanol.

Developing Solvent: CH_2Cl_2 : EtOAC : MeOH : AcOH : H_2O (18 : 3 : 8 : 2 : 2)

Appropriate amount of sample and reference solutions werespotted on the silica gel GF254 plate with microcapillary, developed with prepared developing solvent. Observe the spots exposing the plate to either UV light or iodine, then sprinkle 15% sulphuric acid ethanol solution, heat plate by electric hair-drier, show red to beige color.

6.4 Identification of 2, 3, 5, 4'-stilbene glucoside HPLC Chromatography

Chromatogrphic column: TOSOH TSK gel OSD-100V column (4.6mm × 250mm, 5 μm)

Mobile phase: Acetonitrile-water (25 : 75)

Detection wavelength: 320 nm.

Flow rate: 1.0 ml/min.

Column temperature: 25℃.

Accurately weight 2mg reference and sample of 2, 3, 5, 4'-stilbene glucoside, then dissolve in 50% ethanol to get stock solution, containing 200 μg/ml reference and sample respectively. The stock solutions are filtered through a syringes filter (0.45m μ), 10 μl of aliquots were subjected to HPLC, and determined by the above proposed HPLC-UV conditions. Record the chromatograms, show chromatographic peaks of reference and sample at 7.882 min respectively.

6.3.3 Identified by spectral data (See them in Chinese part.)

7. Notices

7.1 Prefer to use Polygoni multiflori Radix as experimental material, for the lower content of stilbene glucoside of Polygoni Multiflori Radix Praeparata.

7.2 Not to exceed 60℃ when evaporating solvent from the sample silica gel on a water bath, and keep stiring to avoid sample losing.

7.3 Not to elute too fast when subjecting to silica gel column chromatography. It's much better when the amount of elution within 30~60min equals to the weight of stationary.

7.4 2, 3, 5, 4'-stilbene glucoside will be eluted from the second tube generally, note to examine the existence of stilbene glucoside by using the method described above during the experiment.

8. Questions

1. What's the difference in physicochemical properties between stilbene glucoside and anthraquinones? How to identify them?

2. Brief the principle and application of silica gel absorption chromatography?

实验十一　陈皮挥发油的提取与鉴定

一、简介

陈皮为芸香科植物橘 *Citrus reticulata* Blanco 及其栽培变种的干燥成熟果皮，为理气健脾，燥湿化痰的中药。

陈皮挥发油具有刺激性祛痰作用，对胃肠道有温和的刺激作用，能促进消化液分泌和

扫码"学一学"

排除肠内积气，对肺炎双球菌、甲型链球菌等有很强的抑制作用。

陈皮含挥发油 1.5% ~2%，其中主要成分为右旋柠檬酸（约 80% 以上）。

二、目的

掌握挥发油的一般提取和鉴定方法。

三、原理

挥发油与水不相混溶，加热后，当二者蒸气压总和与大气压相等时，溶液开始沸腾，继续加热则挥发油可随水蒸气蒸馏出来。因此，含挥发油的中草药可以利用水蒸气蒸馏法提取其中挥发油。

四、仪器与试剂

1. **仪器** 挥发油提取器，圆底烧瓶（1000 ml），阿贝折光仪，三角瓶（25 ml），烧杯（100 ml），冷凝管。

2. **试剂** 陈皮，硅胶 G 薄层板，石油醚，乙酸乙酯，2% 高锰酸钾溶液，对照品柠檬烯，无水硫酸钠。

五、操作

1. **提取** 称取陈皮粉 100g，置于 1000ml 圆底烧瓶中，加蒸馏水浸过药面，振荡混合，连接挥发油测定器与回流冷凝管。直火回流至测定器中油量不再增加，静置，分层，开启测定器下端活塞，使油层下降至其上端与"0"线平齐，读取挥发油体积，计算百分含量，缓缓放出水分，接收挥发油，加入无水硫酸钠干燥，密闭保存。

2. **鉴定**

（1）记录陈皮挥发油色泽，气味。

（2）测定折光率。

（3）将挥发油滴于滤纸上，加温烘烤，观察油斑是否消失。

（4）薄层色谱

样品：自提陈皮挥发油。

标准品：柠檬烯。

色谱板：硅胶 G 薄层板。

展开剂：石油醚 – 乙酸乙酯（9：21）。

显色剂：2% 高锰酸钾水溶液。

3. **GC – MS 法鉴定**

（1）**仪器** TRACE GC&DSQ 气 – 质联用分析仪（美国 Thermo Finnigan 公司）。

（2）**气相色谱 – 质谱条件** 色谱柱：DB – 5 毛细管柱（30m×0.25m×0.25μm）。电离方式：EI 源。电子能量：70eV。质量范围（m/z）：20 ~500 amu。柱室温度：初始温度 70℃，保持 1min 后，以 4℃/min 速率升至 250℃（保持 10min）。载气：高纯氦气，恒流模式，流速 0.8 ml/min。分流进样，分流比 50：1；进样口温度 270℃，离子源温度 250℃，传输线温度 250℃。

（3）**陈皮挥发油成分分析** 采用 GC – MS 联用技术，对陈皮挥发油进行分析，鉴定了挥发油中主要的 5 个成分，见表 2 - 5。得到各成分的质谱图，直接用该机的数据系统进行检索（谱库），并用标准图谱比较，确定其成分。这 5 个成分的变化在一定程度上可以代表陈皮挥发油成分的变化情况。

表 2 - 5　陈皮中主要的挥发性成分

序号	化学名	分子量	分子式	含量（%）
1	α - 蒎烯	136	$C_{10}H_{16}$	0.70
2	β - 蒎烯	136	$C_{10}H_{16}$	1.12
3	（+）- 4 - 蒈烯	136	$C_{10}H_{16}$	0.16
4	D - 柠檬烯	136	$C_{10}H_{16}$	94.67
5	γ - 松油烯	136	$C_{10}H_{16}$	3.35

六、思考题

1. 挥发油的贮藏应当注意什么？
2. 挥发油的提取还有什么方法？

扫码"练一练"

Experiment Ⅺ　Extraction and Identification of Essential Oil in Citri Reticulatae Pericarpium

1. Introductions

Pericarpium Citri Reticulatae is dried ripe peel of *Citrus reticulata* Blanco, which belongs to Rutaceae family. It is a kind of traditional Chinese medicines, which has effect of regulating qi, strengthening spleen, drying the wetness-evil and eliminating phlegm.

Essential oil has stimulating effect of expelling phlegm and gentle effect on gastrointestinal tract. It can promote digestive juice to secrete and evacuate accumulation of gas in the intestines. It also has depressant effect on pneumococci and alpha streptococcus *etc.*

Pericarpium Citri Reticulatae contains 1.5% ~ 2% essential oil, whose essential component is dextral citric acid (above 80%).

2. Purposes

Learn the extraction, identification method of essential oil.

3. Principles

Essential oil can't mingle with water. Solution starts to boil, when vapor pressure of them equals to atmospheric pressure. Continue to heat, essential oil can follow water vapor to distill out. Therefore, Chinese Herbal containing essential oil can be extracted with this method.

4. Apparatus and Reagents

4.1 Apparatus

Essential oil extractor, round-bottomed flask (1000ml), Abbe refractometer, triangular flask

（25ml），beakers（100ml），condensing tube

4. 2 Reagents

Pericarpium Citri Reticulatae（100g），silica gel G，CMC，petroleum ether，acetic ether，2% Potassium Permanganate，reference limonene，Anhydrous Sodium Sulfate

5. Procedure

5. 1 Extraction

Place 100g of Chenpi crude powder into a 1000ml round bottomed flask，then distill water running the surface of drug. After mixing sufficiently，connect essential oil extractor with reflux condensing tube. Heat directly until essential oil in the analyser doesn't increase. Cool and demix the essential oil，then open the analyser piston until essential oil level to "0" and read the essential oil and calculate percentage content. Expel the water slowly and get essential oil. At last，dry with anhydrous sodium sulfate and store close tightly.

5. 2 Identification

5. 2. 1 Recording color and smell of essential oil of Pericarpium Citri Reticulatae.

5. 2. 2 Measuring refractive index.

5. 2. 3 Drop the essential oil on the filter paper and bake，observe the oil spot.

5. 2. 4 TLC

Sample：Extracted essential oil

Reference sample：Limonene

Adsorbent：Silica gel TLC

Developing Solvent：PE – EtOAc（9：21）

Color developing reagent：2% $KMnO_4$

5. 3 GC – MS

5. 3. 1 Apparatus

TRACE GC&DSQ GC/MS（Thermo Finnigan，American）

5. 3. 2 Conditions of GC – MS

Column：DB – 5 capillary column（30m × 0. 25m × 0. 25μm）. Ionization style：EI. Electron energy：70ev. Mass range（m/z）：20 ~ 500 amu. Column temperature：initiating temperature 70℃，rising the temperature to 250℃（keeping 10min）at 4℃ per minute rate after remaining one minute. Carrier gas：N_2，permanent flow style，0. 8ml/min；split stream injection，split ratio 50：1；injection temperature：270℃，ion source temperature：250℃，transmission line temperature：250℃.

5. 3. 3 Analyzing the constituents

The essential oil was analyzed with GC-MS method. The five components were identified（Table 2 – 5）. Obtaining every compound's MS chart，and retrieve with its data system（spectral library），and compare them with standard spectrogram，determine the components. The difference of the five components can represent the change of the essential oil from Chenpi in some way.

Table 2 – 5　The main volatility constituents in Chenpi

NO	Name	M. W.	Formula	Yield（%）
1	α-Pinene	136	$C_{10}H_{16}$	0.70
2	β-Pinene	136	$C_{10}H_{16}$	1.12
3	（ + ）-4-Carene	136	$C_{10}H_{16}$	0.16
4	D-Limonene	136	$C_{10}H_{16}$	94.67
5	γ-Terpinene	136	$C_{10}H_{16}$	3.35

6. Questions

6.1 What should be noticed when storage essential oil?

6.2 What are the other extraction methods of essential oil?

实验十二　穿心莲内酯的提取、分离和鉴定及亚硫酸氢钠加成物的制备

扫码"学一学"

一、简介

穿心莲为爵床科穿心莲属植物穿心莲 *Andrographis paniculata*（Burm. f. ）Nees 的全草或叶。味苦，性寒，具清热解毒、凉血、消肿、燥湿的功效。穿心莲中含有多种二萜类化合物，其中含量较高的有穿心莲内酯（穿心莲乙素，andrographolides）、新穿心莲内酯（穿心莲丙素，neo-andrographolide）、去氧穿心莲内酯（穿心莲甲素，deoxyandrographolide）等，前两者是穿心莲抗菌消炎的主要有效成分。穿心莲还含有穿心莲烷、甾醇类、黄酮类、甾体、皂苷、糖类、叶绿素和缩合鞣质等类型的化学成分。目前临床上以穿心莲为君药的中成药有 10 余种，包括片剂、注射剂、滴鼻液等，用于治疗急性菌痢、肠胃炎、感冒发热、咽喉炎、尿路感染等。

穿心莲内酯磺化物为穿心莲内酯的衍生物，是经穿心莲内酯与亚硫酸氢钠加成反应制得的水溶性亚硫酸盐，其名称为 14 – 脱羟 – 13 – 脱氢穿心莲内酯 – 12 – 磺酸钠盐，在临床上具有清热解毒，止咳止痢，抗菌消炎作用，用于细菌性痢疾、肺炎、急性扁桃体炎、腮腺炎、喉炎及上呼吸道感染等疾病，目前已有针剂、粉针及冻干粉针等制品。

二、目的

1. 掌握提取、分离穿心莲中穿心莲内酯的方法。

2. 掌握穿心莲内酯的理化性质及鉴定方法。

3. 熟悉穿心莲内酯亚硫酸氢钠加成物的制备方法。

三、原理

1. 穿心莲内酯为白色方棱形或片状结晶（乙醇或甲醇），熔点为 230～231℃，无臭，味苦。易溶于沸乙醇，微溶于甲醇或乙醇，极微溶于三氯甲烷，几乎不溶于水或乙醚。因此，可用乙醇回流提取得到粗总二萜类化合物，然后经乙醇重结晶得到纯品。

2. 穿心莲中含有大量叶绿素，可用活性炭脱色法除去叶绿素杂质。活性炭（acticar-

bon）是一种黑色粉状、粒状或丸状的无定形具有多孔的吸附剂，主要成分为碳，还含少量氧、氢、硫、氮、氯。活性炭具有微晶结构，微晶排列完全不规则，晶体中有微孔、过渡孔、大孔，从而使其具有较大的内表面，比表面积为 $500 \sim 1700$ m²/g，有很强的吸附性能，可用于油脂、饮料、食品、饮用水的脱色、脱味，气体分离、溶剂回收和空气调节，用作催化剂载体和防毒面具的吸附剂。

3. 利用穿心莲内酯结构中具有双键及醇羟基可分别发生酯化、脱水、成盐反应获得其衍生物。

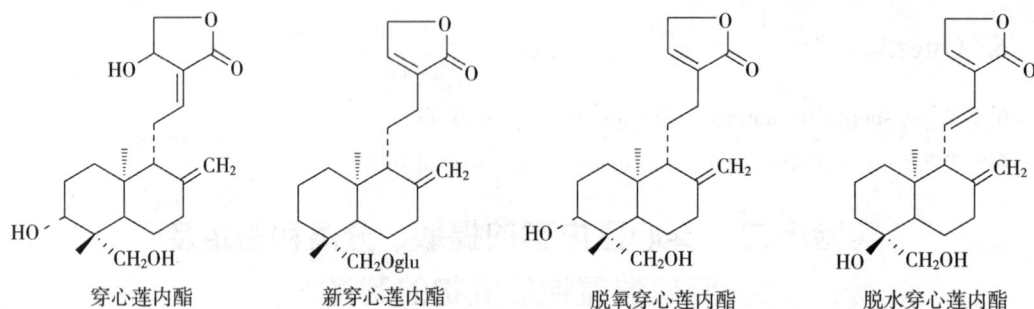

穿心莲内酯　　　　　新穿心莲内酯　　　　　脱氧穿心莲内酯　　　　　脱水穿心莲内酯

四、仪器与试剂

1. **仪器**　烧杯（100 ml，500 ml），圆底烧瓶（50 ml，250 ml，1000 ml），抽滤瓶（250 ml），冷凝管，紫外灯，展开缸，点样毛细管，旋转蒸发仪。

2. **试剂与药品**　乙醇（C. P.），活性炭（C. P.），三氯甲烷（C. P.），亚硫酸氢钠（A. P.）。

五、展开剂及对照品

1. **展开剂**　三氯甲烷 – 甲醇 – 正丁醇（2∶2∶1）。
2. **对照品**　穿心莲内酯。

六、操作

1. 穿心莲内酯的提取与纯化

（1）提取

①渗漉法　取穿心莲粗粉 100 g，加 1.5 倍量 95% 乙醇，放置 30 min，装入渗漉筒内，加 95% 乙醇至液面高过药粉 1～2 cm，浸泡 24 h 后开始渗漉，收集 10 倍量的渗漉液（V/W），将渗漉液减压回收至 400 ml 左右，即为内酯类成分总提取液。

②回流提取法　取穿心莲粗粉 100 g，置于 1000 ml 圆底烧瓶中，加 400 ml 80% 乙醇加热回流提取 1.5 h，用纱布过滤。药渣加 300 ml 80% 乙醇重复提取一次，合并 2 次提取液，浓缩至 300 ml 左右，即为内酯类成分总提取液。

③冷浸法　取穿心莲粗粉 100 g，加 10 倍量 90% 乙醇，室温浸渍 4 天，提取 2 次，合并 2 次提取液，浓缩至 300 ml 左右，即为内酯类成分总提取液。

（2）脱色　取上述内酯类成分总浓缩液，加入原料量 20%（W/V）的活性炭，加热回流 30 min，过滤，并用少量热乙醇洗涤滤渣 2 次，合并滤液和洗涤液，减压浓缩至 15 ml 左右，放置析晶，得穿心莲内酯粗品。称重，计算得率。

（3）分离精制

1）丙酮法 将穿心莲内酯粗品，加 40 倍量丙酮，加热回流 10 min，过滤，不溶物再加 20 倍量丙酮，加热回流 10 min，过滤，合并 2 次滤液，滤液减压浓缩至溶液的三分之一，滤液放置使结晶析出，滤取结晶，得精制穿心莲内酯。干燥称重，计算得率。

2）三氯甲烷法 将穿心莲内酯粗品，加 5 倍量三氯甲烷，振摇，冷浸放置 1h（或加入 3 倍量三氯甲烷回流 10 min），过滤，将不溶物用热三氯甲烷洗涤 2 次，50℃干燥，再加入 15 倍量 95% 乙醇，加热回流溶解，趁热过滤，滤液减压浓缩至半，放冷析晶，抽滤得精制穿心莲内酯。称重，计算得率。

2. 穿心莲内酯亚硫酸氢钠衍生物的制备 该衍生物为白色至类白色无定形粉末，m. p. 226～227 ℃（液化并分解），微具苦味，具有引湿性，易溶于水，可溶于甲醇或乙醇，微溶于三氯甲烷。

（1）反应原理

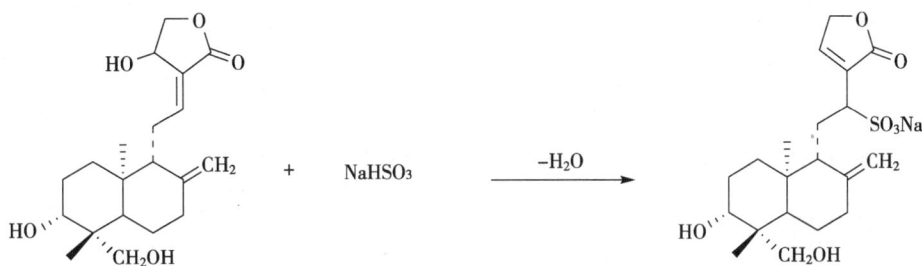

（2）反应工艺 称取精制穿心莲内酯 0.5 g，置于 50 ml 圆底烧瓶中，加 95% 乙醇 5 ml 及适量的 4% 亚硫酸氢钠水溶液，加热回流 30 min。移入蒸发皿中，置水浴上蒸发至无醇味。然后加 5 ml 水溶液溶解，冷却，过滤，滤液用少量三氯甲烷洗涤 3 次，水层置水浴上浓缩至干。残渣加 95% 乙醇 15 ml，滤除不溶物，乙醇溶液减压浓缩得白色粉末，即得穿心莲内酯亚硫酸氢钠加成物。称重，计算反应得率。（注：穿心莲内酯与亚硫酸氢钠加成摩尔比为 1∶1。但是，由于亚硫酸氢钠不稳定，含量易降低，故需新鲜配制，且要求该试剂含量在 95% 以上，并按 100% 换算成实际需要量，因此，实验室制备时宜稍多加亚硫酸氢钠的溶液。）

3. 穿心莲内酯的鉴定

（1）呈色反应

① 异羟肟酸铁反应 取穿心莲内酯结晶少许，加乙醇 1 ml 溶解，加 7% 盐酸羟胺甲醇溶液 2～3 滴，加 10% 氢氧化钾甲醇溶液 1～2 滴使呈碱性，于水浴上加热 2 min，放冷，加稀盐酸使呈酸性，加 1% 三氯化铁试液 1～2 滴，混匀，呈紫红色。

② Legal 反应 取穿心莲内酯结晶少许，加乙醇 1 ml 使溶解，加 0.3% 亚硝酰铁氰化钠溶液 2 滴，10% 氢氧化钠溶液 1 滴，呈紫色。

③ Kedde 反应 取穿心莲内酯结晶少许，加乙醇 1 ml 溶解，加 Kedde 试剂 2 滴，呈紫色。

（2）色谱法鉴别

薄层板：硅胶 G 薄层板。

样品溶液：自制的穿心莲内酯及穿心莲内酯亚硫酸氢钠加成物少量，以适量乙醇溶解。

对照品溶液：穿心莲内酯对照品少量，以适量乙醇溶解。

展开剂：①三氯甲烷－甲醇（9∶1），②三氯甲烷－甲醇－正丁醇（2∶2∶1）。

用毛细管各吸取样品和对照品溶液适量，点于薄层板上，用上述展开剂展开。展开剂吹干后，喷 Kedde 试剂，加热显色。

4. 穿心莲内酯的光谱数据

UV（MeOH）：λmax, nm（ε）：207（sh, 18 095），224（22 447）

ESI-MS（＋）m/z：373［M＋Na］$^+$，389［M＋K］$^+$，723［2M＋Na］$^+$，ESI-MS（－）m/z：349［M-H］$^-$，331［M-H-H$_2$O］$^-$

^{1}H-NMR（C$_5$D$_5$N）δ：0.70（3H, s, 20-CH$_3$），1.51（3H, s, 18-CH$_3$），1.9（signal overlapped）（H-9），2.73（br. t, J＝7.0 Hz, H-11），3.60-3.64（signal overlapped）（2H, br. m, 19-H, H-3），4.43（1H, d, J＝10.5Hz, H-19B），4.50（1H, dd, J＝10.5, 2.5 Hz, H-15），4.60（1H, dd, J＝10.0, 6.0 Hz, H-15B），4.85（1H, br. d, J＝1.0 Hz, H-17A），4.88（1H, br. d, J＝1.0 Hz, H-17B），5.37（br. m, H-14），7.18（1H, td, J＝7.0, 1.5 Hz, H-12）

^{13}C-NMR（C$_5$D$_5$N）：37.4（t, C-1），29.1（t, C-2），80.0（d, C-3），43.3（s, C-4），55.5（d, C-5），24.5（t, C-6），38.3（t, C-7），148.0（s, C-8），56.5（d, C-9），39.3（s, C-10），25.1（t, C-11），147.0（d, C-12），130.3（s, C-13），66.1（d, C-14），75.4（t, C-15），170.7（s, C-16），108.8（t, C-17），23.8（q, C-18），64.2（t, C-19），15.3（q, C-20）

七、思考题

1. 除了用活性炭吸附法去除叶绿素外，还可采用哪些方法去除？

2. 穿心莲总内酯的提取可采用哪些方法？试比较各种方法的优缺点。

3. 根据穿心莲内酯类成分的结构，试判断其极性的强弱，在使用吸附薄层色谱时，穿心莲内酯类成分 R_f 值大小如何？

4. Legal 反应和 Kedde 反应的机制是什么？

Experiment Ⅻ Extraction，Isolation and Identification of Andrographolide and Preparation of the Adduct of Andrographolide with Sodium Hydrogen Sulfite

1. Introductions

Andrographis paniculata（Burm. f.）Nees, with the effectiveness of bitter-cold detoxifying, cooling blood and reducing swelling and dampness, is the herbs of Acanthaceae, and contains diterpenoids. Studies on the chemical composition of *Andrographis paniculata* showed that it is a rich source of diterpenoids including andrographolide, neo-andrographolide, deoxyandrogra pholide, 14-deoxy-11,12-didehydroandrographolide and so on. The former two compounds are the primary components, with the activity of antibacterial effect. Furthermore, steroid alcohols, flavonoids, steroids, saponins, carbohydrates, chlorophyll and condensed tainnin also can be found in Acanthaceae. At present, at least 10 kinds of Chinese formulated products with Acanthaceae as the main composition, including tablet, injection, nasal drops and so on, are used to treat acute bacillary

dysentery, gastroenteritis, influenza-like fever, pharyngitis and urinary tract infection.

Reaction andrographpolide with $NaHSO_3$ and H_2SO_3 produces 14-deoxy-13-dehydroandroa pholide-12 sodium hydrogen sulfite salt, which has good solubility in water, and good effects in curing bacillary dysentery, pneumonia, acute tonsillitis, mumps, laryngitis and upper respiratory tract infection and other diseases.

2. Purposes

2. 1 To learn how to extract, isolate andrographolide.

2. 2 To master the physical and chemical properties and identification method of andrographolide.

2. 3 To grasp the preparation method of the adduct of andrographolide with sodium hydrogen sulfite.

3. Principles

3. 1 Andrographolide, white square prism or crystal (ethanol or methanol), m. p. 230 ~ 231℃, bitter. It is dissolved in boiling ethanol, slightly soluble in methanol or ethanol, very slightly soluble in chloroform, and almost insoluble in water and aether. Therefore, ethanol can be applied as the solvent for the extraction and recrystallization of andrographolides. The structure of andrographolide contains conjugate double bond and hydroxyl groups, so it can be prepared into sulfonating, addition or esterifying.

3. 2 Activated carbon, so called activated charcoal or activated coal, is in the forms of black powder, granule or pellets with a porous amorphous carbon, the main components is carbon, also contain a small amount of oxygen, hydrogen, sulfur, nitrogen and chlorine. Activated carbon has a microcrystalline structure, which is completely in irregular range. There are microbore transition holes and large holes, making it the inner surface has a larger specific surface area of 500 ~ 1700 m^2/g, has a strong adsorption and can be used for oils and fats, beverages, foods, drinking water decolorization, off flavor, gas separation, solvent recovery and air-conditioning, the adsorbent of gas masks and catalyst. Andrographis contains a large amount of chlorophyll, which can be removed by active carbon.

3. 3 Andrographolides contain double bond and alcoholic hydroxyl group, which can esterify, dehydrate and form salt to get derivatives.

4. Apparatus and reagents

4. 1 Apparatus

Beaker (100 ml, 500 ml), round bottom flask (50 ml, 250 ml, 1000 ml), suction flask (250 ml), condenser, UV light, developing chamber for TLC, macrocapillary (1 mm), rotary evaporator.

4. 2 Reagents

Ethanol (C. P.), activated carbon (C. P.), chloroform (C. P.), sodium bisulfite (A. P.).

5. Developing solvents and references

5. 1 Developing solvents

Chloroform：methanol：n-butanol（2：2：1）.

5. 2 References

Andrographolide.

6. Procedures

6. 1 Extraction and purification of andrographolide

6. 1. 1 Extraction

6. 1. 1. 1 Percolation method　Put Andrographitis coarse powder（100 g）into a 500 ml beaker, which contains 1. 5 times volume of 95% to mix it sufficiently, place into a percolator after keeping it for 30 minutes. Then, 95% ethanol is added to the surface of powders for 1 ~ 2cm, and for 24h, then collect 10 times the volume of colature（V/W）, concentrate colature to 400 ml, which is the extract of total lactones.

6. 1. 1. 2 Reflux extraction method　Weigh andrographitis coarse powder（100 g）into 1000ml beaker with 400 ml 80% ethanol then reflux for 1. 5h. Filter the extracting solution with gauze and extract the gruffness with 80% ethanol（300 ml）for 1. 5h again. Combine the extract and concentrate to about 300ml to obtain the total lactones.

6. 1. 1. 3 Cold maceration method　Extract Andrographitis coarse powder（100 g）with 10 times the amount of 90% ethanol in a 1000 ml beaker at room temperature for 4 days, filter to get the extraction solution. Repeat 2 times. The combined extract was concentrated to 300 ml to obtain the total lactones.

6. 1. 2 Decolorization

Add the amount of raw materials 20% of activated carbon to the lactone components of theconcentrated extraction, then heated to recirculate for 30 minutes. Filtering, and washing with a small amount of hot ethanol for 2 times. Combined filtrate and washing solution, concentrated to about 15ml using vacuum rotary evaporation. Lay up till white crystal occurs and filter it. Finally, the crude andrographolide can be obtained. Weigh and calculate the yield.

6. 1. 3 Separation and Purification

6. 1. 3. 1 Acetone method　Crude and rographolide plus 40 times the volume of acetone was heated to reflux for 10 minutes. Filtering. Insolubles plus 20 times the amount of acetone was refluxed for 10 minutes. Filtering. Combine the acetone solution and evaporated to one-third of the volume. Filtrate was placed so that precipitation of leaching crystallization andrographolide was refined. Weigh and calculate the yield.

6. 1. 3. 2 Chloroform method　Add 5 times chloroform to crude andrographolide, shake and cold macerate for 1h（or reflux with 3 times chloroform for 10 min）, filter, extract the insolubles with hot chloroform for 2 times. Drying at 50℃, then dissolve it with 15 times 95% ethanol by refluxing, filter when it is hot, concentrate the filtrate under vacuum condition to a half. Filtrate was placed for crystallization to get refined andrographolide. Weigh and calculate the yield .

6. 2 Preparation of Andrographolide sodium bisulfite adduct

The adduct is white or almost white amorphous powder, m. p. $226 \sim 227\,^\circ\!C$, (liquefaction and decomposition), slightly bitter, easy moist, soluble in water, methanol or ethanol, slightly soluble in chloroform.

6. 2. 1 Principle of reaction

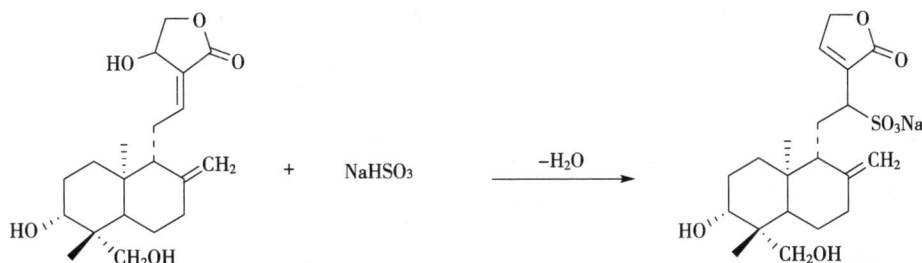

6. 2. 2 The reaction process

Put 0. 5gandrographolide in 50ml flask, add 5ml 95% ethanol and an appropriate amount of 4% sodium bisulfite aqueous solution, reflux for 30min. Then transfer to the evaporating dish and evaporate to no alcohol taste by water-bath. Add 5ml water to dissolve it, cool and filter. Washing the filtrate with a small amount of chloroform for 3 times. Put aqueous layer above water bath to dry. Added 95% ethanol 15ml to residues, filter, condense the ethanol solution to get white power (adduct), weigh and calculate the yield.

(Note: The molar ratio ofandrographolide and sodium bisulfite is 1 : 1. However, because the sodium bisulfite is unstable and easy to reduce the content, so it needs to be prepared freshly with the content over 95% and by 100% converted into the actual requirement, therefore, slightly add more sodium biaulfate solution when prepare the adduct in lab.)

6. 3 Identification of andrographolide

6. 3. 1 Color reaction

6. 3. 1. 1 Ferric hydroxamic acid reaction: Dissolve a little andrographolide with 1ml ethanol, add $2 \sim 3$ drops 7% hydroxylamine hydrochloride/MeOH, then add $1 \sim 2$ drops 10% potassium hydroxide/MeOH to make the solution show basicity, heat the solution by water bath for 2 minitues, then leave it to cool, add diluted hydrochloric acid to make the solution show acidity, add $1 \sim 2$ drop 1% ferric chloride test solution, blend, observe the phenomenon.

6. 3. 1. 2 Legal reaction: Dissolve a little andrographolide with 1ml ethanol, add 2 drops 0. 3% natrium nitroferrocyanatum solution and 1 drop 10% sodium hydroxide solution, observe the phenomenon.

6. 3. 1. 3 Kedde reaction: Dissolve a little andrographolide with 1ml ethanol, add 2 drops Kedde reagent, observe the phenomenon.

6. 3. 2 The chromatography identification

Thin-layer plate: Silica gel G-CMC-Na thin plate.

Sample solution: A small amount self-made andrographolide and andrographolide sodium bisulfite adduct dissolved in appropriate ethanol.

Reference standard: A small amount of reference substance androgrpholide to moderate a ethanol dissolved.

Developing agent：①chloroform-methanol（9：1），②chloroform-methanol-*n*-butanol（2：2：1）.

Appropriate amount of sample and reference solutions are applied with microcapillary, developed by above developing solvents, then the plate are sprayed with Kedde reagent, coloration appears under heat.

6.4 Spectral datas of andrographolide（See them in Chinese part.）

7. Questions

7.1 Which methods can be used to remove chlorophyll except being adsorped by activated carbon?

7.2 Which methods can be used to extract the total lactones in *Andrograghis paniculata* （Burm. f.）Nees? Compare the advantages and disadvantages of different methods.

7.3 Judge the polarities of lacones in *Andrograghis paniculata* （Burm. f.）Nees and thier R_f values of thin-layer chromatography.

7.4 What are the reaction mechanisms of Legal reaction and Kedde reaction?

实验十三　紫杉烷类二萜的提取、分离和鉴定

一、简介

紫杉烷类化合物，包括抗癌药紫杉醇，是从红豆杉属植物中分离到的二萜类化合物。红豆杉最早的化学研究始于 Lucas，1856 年他从其中分离到二萜生物碱类化合物，并命名为Taxine。紫杉醇（taxol）和巴卡亭－Ⅲ（baccatin－Ⅲ）是紫杉烷类化合物中重要且具有代表性的化合物。紫杉醇是一种新型的天然抗肿瘤药物，而巴卡亭－Ⅲ则是紫杉醇的重要的二萜母核部分。

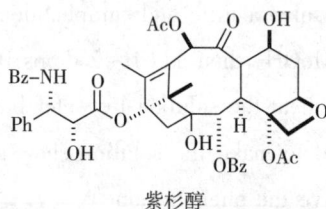

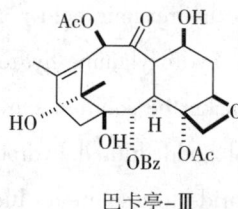

紫杉醇　　　　　　　　　巴卡亭-Ⅲ

二、目的

学习从红豆杉属植物中提取、分离和鉴定紫杉烷二萜类化合物的方法。

三、原理

紫杉烷二萜是一类具有小到中等极性的成分，可用乙醇或甲醇等醇性溶剂提取，通过萃取（三氯甲烷－水）、色谱和重结晶等方法分离纯化；所得产物使用硅胶薄层色谱实验检测，用三氯甲烷和甲醇的混合溶剂展开，香草醛－硫酸溶液喷雾并加热，紫杉烷可显不同颜色的色斑。

四、仪器与试剂

1. 仪器 色谱柱（2 cm×10 cm），分液漏斗（100 ml），旋转蒸发仪，硅胶 G 薄层板（微型），薄层色谱缸（小型），喷雾试剂瓶，锥形瓶（50 ml），电吹风或电热板。

2. 试剂 硅胶（柱色谱规格），环己烷（A. R.），石油醚（A. R.），三氯甲烷（A. R.），二氯甲烷（A. R.），乙醇（A. R.），甲醇（A. R.），5% 香草醛 – 硫酸（硫酸：无水乙醇 =4∶1）喷雾试剂。

五、实验过程

1. 植物材料准备 准备美丽红豆杉即南方红豆杉 *Taxus chinensis* var. *mairei* Cheng et L. K. Fu 或其他种的叶和小枝。说明：红豆杉植物材料应是新鲜的，并经适当干燥及粉碎。

2. 提取 将准备好的植物材料，用乙醇回流提取三次，每次 2 小时。过滤后，滤液于 45℃减压浓缩，得到浸膏。

3. 萃取 浸膏以水混悬后，以适当的有机溶剂（即二氯甲烷、三氯甲烷、己烷、石油醚等）萃取。经三氯甲烷萃取 3 次，三氯甲烷层即可得到富集的紫杉烷。

4. 液相色谱分离 将三氯甲烷溶解的化合物进行常压或低压柱色谱分离，包括正相柱色谱和反相柱色谱。正相柱色谱，通常用硅胶或氧化铝；而反相柱色谱常用 C18 硅胶。柱色谱的过程应使用 TLC 或 HPLC 监测。

5. 薄层鉴定 准备样品溶液，将步骤 4 所得紫杉烷样品溶于少量二氯甲烷（或三氯甲烷）中。并使用硅胶薄层板检测，以三氯甲烷：甲醇（95∶5）溶液展开，用 5% 香草醛 – 硫酸试剂喷雾，105℃加热至样品显色。

6. 重结晶 在振摇和加热条件下，将紫杉烷样品溶于少量乙醇或甲醇中，静置使其析晶。结晶减压滤出，抽干，干燥得纯紫杉烷结晶。

六、巴卡亭Ⅲ的波谱数据

Baccatin Ⅲ：m. p：236～238℃（dec.）；$[\alpha]_D^{25}$：−54（MeOH）

UV（nm）：230（13900），274（1000），282（850）

CI-MS：587 $[M+H]^+$，569，527，509，405，345，123

^{1}H-NMR（400 MHz，CDCl$_3$）δ：5.60（1H，d，$J=7.5$ Hz，H-3），3.86（1H，d，$J=7.3$ Hz，H-2），4.97（1H，d，$J=8.6$ Hz，H-5），2.55（1H，m，6β-H），1.85（1H，m，6α-H），4.45（1H，m，7-H），6.30（1H，s，10-H），4.88（1H，br. t，$J=8.8$ Hz，13-H），2.27（1H，m，14-H），1.08（3H，s，16-H），1.08（3H，s，17-H），2.04（3H，s，18-H），1.65（3H，s，19-H），4.29（1H，d，$J=8.4$ Hz，20β-H），4.13（1H，d，$J=8.4$ Hz，20α-H），2.27（3H，s，4-OCOCH$_3$），2.23（3H，s，10-OCOCH$_3$），8.10（2H，d，$J=7.9$ Hz，*o*-H（BzCOO）），7.46（2H，t，$J=7.8$ Hz，*m*-H（BzCOO）），7.59 [1H，t，$J=7.5$ Hz，*p*-H（BzCOO）]

^{13}C-NMR（100 MHz，CDCl$_3$）：79.1（s，C-1），74.9（d，C-2），46.1（d，3-C），80.8（s，4-C），84.4（d，5-C），35.6（t，6-C），72.3（d，7-C），58.7（s，8-C），204.1（s，9-C），76.2（d，10-C），131.9（s，11-C），146.3（s，12-C），68.0（d，13-C），38.6（t，14-C），42.7（s，15-C），20.9（q，16-C），27.0（q，17-C），15.6（q，18-C），9.4（q，19-C），76.4（t，20-C），

170. 6（s, 4-COCH$_3$）, 171. 3（s, 10-COCH$_3$）, 22. 6（q, 4-COCH$_3$）, 20. 9（q, 10-COCH$_3$）, 167. 1（s, *o*-BzCOO）, 129. 3（s, 1-BzCOO）, 130. 1（d, *o*- BzCOO）, 128. 6（d, *m*- BzCOO）, 133. 7（d, *p*- BzCOO）

七、备注

1. 红豆杉植物材料应是新鲜或经适当干燥的，否则紫杉烷可能在提取前降解。

2. 5%香草醛－硫酸喷雾剂应是新鲜配制，以期得到更好的（显色）效果。

八、实验室操作

1. 红豆杉的热回流提取。

2. 紫杉烷两相萃取（三氯甲烷∶水）。

3. 紫杉烷二萜的薄层色谱鉴定。

4. 紫杉烷的柱色谱分离。

5. 紫杉烷的重结晶。

九、思考题

1. 描述紫杉烷提取和分离的一般过程。

2. 描述在薄层色谱实验中，紫杉烷的色斑在加热时的变色过程。

十、讨论

1. 至今已从红豆杉属植物中分离得到多少种紫杉烷类化合物？

2. 应该如何解决紫杉醇来源有限的问题？

扫码"练一练"

Experiment ⅩⅢ   Extraction，Isolation and Identification of Taxane Diterpenoids

1. Introduction

The taxanes are diterpenoids，isolated from plants of *Taxus* species，that include paclitaxel（taxol），which are used in the treatment of cancer. The first chemical study of a *Taxus* species was carried out by Lucas，who isolated an alkaloidal substance which he named taxine in 1856. The taxane diterpenoids have been reviewed on several previous occasions. Both taxol and baccatin Ⅲ are the important compounds in taxanes. Taxol is a new-type natural anti-cancer drug，and baccatin Ⅲ is the important diterpenoid portion of taxol.

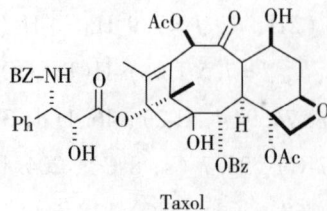

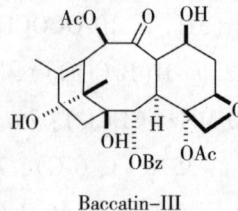

Taxol　　　　　　　Baccatin-Ⅲ

2. Purpose

From this experiment, students will learn how to extract, isolate taxane diterpenoids from Taxus species, and identify them.

3. Principles

Taxane diterpenoids are constituents with moderate to small polarity, which can be extracted with alcoholic solvents such as ethanol or methanol, and purified through partition (between $CHCl_3$ and H_2O), chromatography and recrystalization.

In their silica gel TLC test, developed with a mixture of $CHCl_3$ and MeOH, sprayed with 5% vanillin-H_2SO_4 reagent, and heated, taxanes appeared as different color spots.

4. Apparatus and Reagents

4.1 Apparatus

Small chromatography column ($2cm \times 10cm$), Separatory funnel (100 ml), Rotatory evaporator, SiO_2 GF_{254} TLC plates (micro size), TLC development tank (mini type), Spray reagent bottle, Conical flasks (50 ml), Electric heater or hot plate.

4.2 Reagents

SiO_2 (column chromatography grade), Cyclo-hexanes (A. R.), petroleum ether (A. R.), $CHCl_3$ (A. R.), CH_2Cl_2 (A. R.), EtOH (A. R.), MeOH (A. R.), 5% Vanlllin-H_2SO_4 (H_2SO_4: anhydrous EtOH = 4 : 1) spray reagent.

5. Procedures

5.1 Preparation of Plant material

Needles and twigs, or heart wood of *Taxus chinensis* var. *mairei* Cheng et L. (or other *Taxus* species). Plant material of *Taxus* species should be fresh, properly dried, and grounded.

5.2 Extraction

Well-prepared plant material, mentioned above, was extracted with ethanol three times for 2 hours. Extract is filtered and evaporated under 45℃ in vacuum to remove ethanol, and yield a residue.

5.3 Partition

The residue is partitioned between H_2O and certain organic solvent (e. g. CH_2Cl_2, $CHCl_3$, hexanes, petroleum ether and so on). Through one or more partitions, more concentrated solutions of taxanes can be obtained in CH_2Cl_2 or $CHCl_3$ layer.

5.4 Liquid chromatographic separations

CH_2Cl_2 (or $CHCl_3$) soluble constituents was then submitted to column chromatography isolation under normal, or low pressure. It includes normal phase liquid chromatography (LC) and reverse phase liquid chromatography (RPLC). Usually, silica gel or aluminum oxide was used in LC and C 18-silica in RPLC. The process of column chromatography should be monitored by TLC or HPLC.

5. 5 TLC Identification

Dissolve taxane samples in small amount of CH_2Cl_2 (or $CHCl_3$) to prepare sample solution. The solution is applied to SiO_2 GF_{254} TLC plate, developed with a mixture of $CHCl_3$ and MeOH (95 : 5), sprayed with 5% Vanlllin-H_2SO_4 reagent, heated with a heater, and the taxanes appeared as colored spots.

5. 6 Recrystallization

Dissolve taxane sample into small amount of EtOH or MeOH, while shaking and warming, and let stand for recrystallization. The crystals are filtered under suction, into dryness, and dried to yield pure taxane crystals.

6. Spectral Data of Baccatin Ⅲ

Shown in the Chinese version.

7. Notices

7. 1 Plant material of *Taxus* species should be fresh or properly dried, otherwise taxanes may degrade before extraction.

7. 2 Vanlllin (5%)-H_2SO_4 spray reagent should be new prepared, in order to get better results.

8. Lab assignment

8. 1 Extraction of *Taxus chinensis* var. *mairei* (or other *Taxus* species

8. 2 Partion of taxanes between $CHCl_3$ and H_2O.

8. 3 TLC test of taxanes diterpenoids.

8. 4 Column chromatographic isolation of taxanes.

8. 5 Recrytallization of taxanes.

9. Questions

9. 1 Generally describe the process of taxanes' extraction and isolation.

9. 2 Describe the changing process of the color spots of the taxanes, in it's TLC test, during heating.

10. Discussion

10. 1 How many kinds of taxanes have been isolated and identified from *Taxus species*?

10. 2 The source of toxol is not enough, how can we get more?

实验十四　白头翁皂苷的提取、分离和鉴定

一、简介

白头翁是毛茛科白头翁属植物白头翁 *Pulsatilla chinensis* （Bge）Regel 的干燥根，主治热

毒血痢、鼻衄、阿米巴痢等疾病。有效成分为三萜皂苷，主要为白头翁皂苷 B_4（anemoside B_4），其母核为羽扇豆烷型五环三萜。

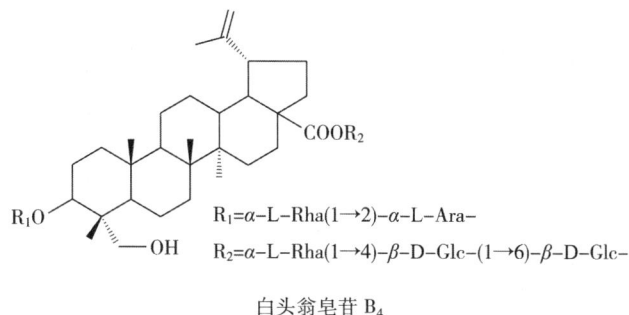

$R_1=\alpha\text{-L-Rha}(1\rightarrow2)\text{-}\alpha\text{-L-Ara-}$
$R_2=\alpha\text{-L-Rha}(1\rightarrow4)\text{-}\beta\text{-D-Glc-}(1\rightarrow6)\text{-}\beta\text{-D-Glc-}$

白头翁皂苷 B_4

二、目的

1. 掌握提取、分离和纯化白头翁总皂苷的方法。
2. 掌握大孔吸附树脂的使用方法。
3. 熟悉三萜皂苷的鉴别反应。

三、原理

白头翁皂苷是大极性成分，能被醇性溶剂（如甲醇、乙醇等）提取及通过大孔吸附树脂得到纯化。含有主要皂苷成分可以通过与标准品的比较加以确定。

大孔吸附树脂是一种不含交换基团的具有大孔结构的高分子吸附剂，是一种亲脂性物质，具有各种不同的表面性质，依靠分子中的亲脂键，偶极离子及氢键的作用，可以有效地吸附具有不同化学性质的各种类型化合物，同时也容易解吸附。

大孔吸附树脂可按极性强弱分为极性、中极性和非极性三种。如 D101 型大孔树脂，为非极性吸附树脂，其结构是聚 2 - 甲基苯乙烯，具有选择性好，吸附容量大，再生处理简单，机械强度高等优点，应用广泛。大孔树脂具有反相色谱和分子筛双重原理，对大分子亲水性成分吸附力弱，对亲脂性物质吸附力强，适用于亲水性和中等极性物质的分离。可除去混合物中的糖和低极性小分子有机物，被分离组分间极性差别越大，分离效果越好。一般用水、含水甲醇或乙醇、丙酮（10%、20%．V/V）洗脱，最后用浓醇或丙酮洗脱，再生时用甲醇或乙醇洗涤即可。

四、仪器与试剂

1. **仪器**　圆底烧瓶（500 ml），烧杯（500 ml），三角瓶（500 ml），索氏提取器，冷凝管，色谱柱（3 cm × 40 cm），TLC 展开缸，水浴锅，旋转蒸发仪。

2. **试剂**　白头翁根，白头翁皂苷 B_4 标准品，D101 型大孔吸附树脂，硅胶薄层板，95%乙醇、乙醚，BAW 试剂，10%硫酸显色液。

五、操作

1. **大孔树脂的预处理**　取 D101 型大孔树脂 100 g，于 500 ml 索氏提取器中，用300 ml 95%乙醇回流 2.5 小时，待回流液 1 份加 3 份水无浑浊时，取出树脂沥干乙醇转入蒸馏水中，浸泡待用。

2. 白头翁总皂苷的提取　取 50 g 白头翁药材，加 200 ml 95% 乙醇回流 1.5 小时，过滤，再重复提取 1 次。合并滤液，回收乙醇至 10 ml，加乙醚 30 ml 沉淀，倒出上清液，过滤，沉淀用水溶解，加少量活性炭脱色、过滤，滤液为白头翁总皂苷部分。

3. 色谱分离　取 3 cm × 40 cm 的玻璃色谱柱，下端垫上棉花，湿法装入 60 g 大孔树脂，上端再加少许棉花，取总皂苷上柱，用水 200 ml 洗，再分别用 20%，50%，95% 乙醇各 200 ml 洗脱，至洗脱流份中不含皂苷，收集各洗脱液流份。

六、皂苷的鉴定方法

1. 白头翁皂苷的薄层色谱检测

样品：洗脱液 20%、50% 和 95% 乙醇部分各流份取 10 ml 减压浓缩至 2 ml 点样。

对照品：白头翁皂苷 B_4。

薄层板：硅胶 G 薄层板。

展开剂：BAW（正丁醇：醋酸：水 = 4：1：1）。

显色剂：10% 硫酸液 105℃ 显色。

2. 光谱鉴别法

白头翁皂苷 B_4：白色粉末，熔点 182～184 ℃，溶于吡啶

IR（ν_{max}，KBr，cm^{-1}）：4300，1730，1640

MS（m/z）：1243，1221，1075，943，927，913，781，773，751，619，605，473，455，437

^{1}H-NMR（C_5D_5N）δ：1.77（3H，s，H-30），1.23（3H，s，H-27），1.12（3H，s，H-26），1.04（3H，s，H-25），0.96（3H，s，H-24），4.92，4.75（each 1H，brs，H_2-29），1.71（3H，d，J = 6.0 Hz，6-H_3 of rha），1.78（3H，d，J = 5.5 Hz，6'-H_3 of rha），5.21（1H，d，J = 7.5 Hz，H-1 of ara），5.91（1H，brs，1'-H of rha），6.28（1H，brs，1-H of rha），6.42（1H，d，J = 8.0 Hz，1'-H of glc），5.02（1H，d，J = 8.0 Hz，1''-H of glc）

^{13}C-NMR（C_5D_5N）δ：39.3（C-1），26.2（C-2），81.3（C-3），43.5（C-4），47.9（C-5），18.3（C-6），34.4（C-7），41.3（C-8），51.1（C-9），37.1（C-10），21.4（C-11），26.2（C-12），38.5（C-13），42.9（C-14），31.0（C-15），32.3（C-16），57.1（C-17），47.4（C-18），50.0（C-19），150.9（C-20），30.2（C-21），36.9（C-22），64.3（C-23），13.5（C-24），16.9（C-25），16.5（C-26），14.9（C-27），175.1（C-28），109.9（C-29），19.5（C-30），3-O-Ara：103.9（C-1'），76.2（C-2'），73.3（C-3'），68.4（C-4'），64.3（C-5'），Rha：101.4（C-1''），72.2（C-2''），72.5（C-3''），73.8（C-4''），69.7（C-5''），18.3（C-6''），28-O-Glc：95.2（C-1'），73.7（C-2'），78.4（C-3'），70.9（C-4'），76.4（C-5'），69.5（C-6'），Glc：104.6（C-1''），75.1（C-2''），76.8（C-3''），78.8（C-4''），77.7（C-5''），61.5（C-6''），Rha：102.4（C-1'''），71.9（C-2'''），72.5（C-3'''），73.8（C-4'''），70.2（C-5'''），18.3（C-6'''）

七、思考题

1. 白头翁总皂苷的提取、分离的原理是什么？
2. 大孔吸附色谱分离原理是什么？

Experiment ⅩⅣ　Extraction, Isolation and Identification of Saponins from Pulsatillae Radix

1. Introduction

Radic pulsatillae, the roots of *Pulsatilla chinensis* (Bge) Regel, is a very important traditional Chinese medicines. It has been used as an anti-amoebiasis, anti-inflammatory, and anti-spasmodic agent. The saponins were been thought to be the main activie substance of of *P. chinensis*, including anemoside B_4, etc.

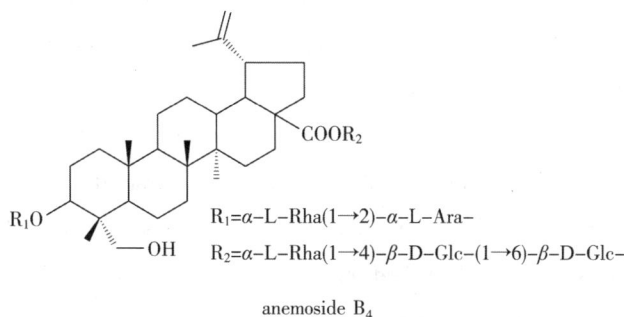

$$R_1 = \alpha\text{-L-Rha}(1\rightarrow2)\text{-}\alpha\text{-L-Ara-}$$
$$R_2 = \alpha\text{-L-Rha}(1\rightarrow4)\text{-}\beta\text{-D-Glc-}(1\rightarrow6)\text{-}\beta\text{-D-Glc-}$$

anemoside B_4

2. Purpose

2.1 Master how to extract, purify and identify the total saponins from Pulsatillae radix.

2.2 Master how to use the macroporous adsorption resin.

2.2 Familiar with the identify reactions of triterpenoid saponins.

3. Principle

Saponins from Radic pulsatillae are polarity constituents, so it could be extracted with alcoholic solvents such as methanol and ethanol, and purified by a D101 macroporous adsorption resin column. The main saponins (anemoside B_4) could be identified by direct comparison of R_f values with authentic sample.

Macroporous adsorption resin is an artificially synthetic polymer adsorbent which has multi hole three dimensifon structures. It is a new type resin developed from application of ion exchange and other adsorbent. The principle of its wok is physical adsorption by way of the Van Der Waals force between itself and adsorbed molecules and through its huge ratio surface. It has very strong adsorbing ability to those molecules with similar structure such as aroma annular chemical compound. The process of using synthetic adsorption extraction make solvent to be reduced and safer than other adsorption.

4. Apparatus and reagents

4.1 Apparatus

Round-bottom flask (500 ml), beaker (500 ml), conical flask (500 ml), Soxhlet's apparatus, condenser pipe, chromatography column (3 cm × 40 cm), TLC development tank, water-bath, rotary evaporator.

4. 2 Reagents

Crude powder of the roots of *Pulsatilla chinensis*, anemoside B_4, D 101 macroporous adsorption resin, SiO_2 G TLC plates, 95 % EtOH, Ethyl ether(A. R.), BAW, 10% H_2SO_4.

5. Procedures

5. 1 Pretreatment of macroporous adsorption resin

Put D101 macroporous adsorption resin (100 g) into Soxhlet extractor (500 ml), add 95% EtOH (300 ml) under refluxing for 2. 5 hours. The resin rinsed in distilled water and store up with distilled water till no deposition appear in the mixture solution (reflux solution : water = 1 : 3).

5. 2 Extraction of the Total Saponins

The powdered roots of *P. chinensis* (50 g) are extracted with 95% EtOH (200 ml) under reflux for 1. 5 hours. Filter and transfer the solution, and then extract the residue as the same method again, filter. Combine the filtrate and evaporate in vacuum to remove ethanol to 10 ml, add ethyl ether (30 ml) keep the solution undisturbed for 5 ~ 10 minutes, pour out the upper clear solution, filter it, deposition dissolved in water, add a small amount of activated charcoal, filter it, the filtrate is total saponins of Pulsatillae radix.

5. 3 Column chromatography separation

Force a small piece of glass wool down the column, slowly fill the column with macroporous adsorption resin (60 g), add a piece of glass wool cover with macroporous adsorption resin. The obtained total saponins is chromatographed on macroporous adsorption resin column, using 200 ml H_2O, 20% EtOH, 50% EtOH, 95% EtOH as eluents. Detecting the eluting solution with TLC method, collect the same fraction.

6. General identification forsaponins

6. 1 TLC Identification

Samples: put each of fractions 20% EtOH-water, 50% EtOH-water, and 95% EtOH-water 10 ml, concentrated to 2 ml by rotary evaporation.

Standard: anemoside B_4.

TLC plate: silica gel G.

Solvent system: BAW (*n*-BuOH : HAc : H_2O = 4 : 1 : 1).

Detection system: 10 % H_2SO_4, dry them under an applied vacuum at 105 ℃.

6. 2 Identified by spectral data (See them in Chinese part.)

7. Questions

1. Generally describe the principle of extracting and isolating of saponins from *P. chinensis*.

2. Generally describe the usage principle of macroporous adsorption resin.

实验十五　齐墩果酸的提取、分离和鉴定

一、简介

齐墩果酸属于五环三萜类化合物，以游离体和配糖体的形式存在于多种植物中，在女贞子中含量可达到8%。女贞子为木犀科植物女贞 *Ligustrum lucidum* Ait. 的干燥成熟果实。药理研究证明齐墩果酸有减少转氨酶的作用，对四氯化碳引起的大鼠急性肝损伤有明显的保护作用，临床上已用于治疗急性黄疸型肝炎，对慢性肝炎也有一定的疗效。

二、目的

1. 掌握五环三萜类化合物的提取、分离方法。
2. 熟悉五环三萜类化合物的主要化学性质。
3. 掌握应用薄层色谱鉴定齐墩果酸的方法。

三、原理

齐墩果酸为白色针晶（乙醇），m. p. 309～310℃，分子式 $C_{30}H_{48}O_3$，分子量456.71。无臭，无味；可溶于甲醇、乙醇、苯、乙醚、丙酮和三氯甲烷，几乎不溶于水。

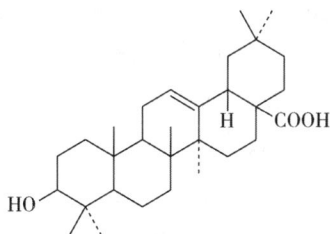

齐墩果酸

四、仪器与试剂

1. **仪器**　烧杯（1000 ml），圆底烧瓶（250 ml），量筒（100 ml），锥形瓶（500 ml），布氏漏斗，抽滤瓶，冷凝管，循环水泵，蒸馏头，牛角管，展开缸，点样毛细管（1 mm），电炉，烘箱，水浴锅，喷瓶。

2. **试剂**　95%工业乙醇，95%乙醇（分析纯），6 mol/L盐酸，滤纸（5 cm×8 cm），硅胶 G 薄层层析板。

五、展开剂、显色剂及对照品

1. **展开剂**　石油醚－乙酸乙酯（3∶1）（1滴乙酸），环己烷－乙酸乙酯（8∶2）。
2. **显色剂**　5%香草醛－浓硫酸溶液。
3. **对照品**　齐墩果酸。

六、操作

1. 齐墩果酸的提取和纯化

（1）提取　称取干燥女贞子果实 50 g，加 300 ml 水浸泡 4 d。水浸液弃去，药材再加 300 ml 水煮沸 20 min，浆状汤弃去。将药渣皮仁分离，种仁、种皮弃去，得到果皮果肉（皮渣）。皮渣置烘箱中 80～90℃ 干燥。干燥后将皮渣粉碎，用 50 ml 95% 乙醇（约 10 倍量）加热回流提取 2 次，每次 30 min。药渣弃去，合并两次乙醇提取液。提取液浓缩至一半体积，加水（1∶1，体积比）混合，用 6mol/L 盐酸调 pH 1，放置过夜，析晶。抽滤得齐墩果酸粗品。干燥称重，计算得率。

（2）重结晶　齐墩果酸粗品 1 g，用 90% 乙醇加热溶解，趁热抽滤，放置使结晶析出，得精制齐墩果酸，干燥称重，计算得率。或者齐墩果酸粗品 1 g，用正己烷 - 乙醇（1∶1）溶解，过滤，放置使析出结晶，得精制齐墩果酸，干燥称重，计算得率。

2. 齐墩果酸的鉴定

（1）呈色反应　取齐墩果酸少许置试管中，加酸酐 1ml，溶解后，沿试管壁加浓硫酸数滴，在两液层交界处，出现紫红色环。

（2）薄层鉴定

薄层板：硅胶 G 薄层板

样品：自制齐墩果酸少量，加 95% 乙醇加热溶解。

对照品：齐墩果酸精制品少量，加 95% 乙醇加热溶解。

展开剂：石油醚 - 乙酸乙酯（3∶1）（1 滴乙酸）或者环己烷 - 乙酸乙酯（8∶2）。

用毛细管各吸取样品和对照品溶液适量，点于硅胶板上，用上述展开剂展开。展开剂挥干后，喷香草醛 - 浓硫酸溶液，置烘箱中 105℃ 烘烤 5 min 显色。

（3）光谱法鉴别

IR $(\nu_{max}^{KBr}, cm^{-1})$:3440（OH），1700（C＝O），1600（C＝C）

EI-MS (m/z) :455 $[M-H]^-$

^{1}H-NMR（400 MHz，C_5D_5N）δ:5.27（1H，br. s，H-12），3.22（1H，dd，J = 5.7，10.1 Hz，H-3），3.29（1H，m，H-18），0.87，0.93，0.99，1.01，1.23，1.27，1.83（each 3H，s，7×CH_3）

^{13}C-NMR（100 MHz，C_5D_5N）δ：38.9（C-1），28.1（C-2），78.1（C-3），39.4（C-4），55.8（C-5），18.8（C-6），33.2（C-7），39.7（C-8），48.1（C-9），37.4（C-10），23.7（C-11），122.5（C-12），144.8（C-13），42.1（C-14），28.3（C-15），23.8（C-16），46.7（C-17），42.0（C-18），46.6（C-19），30.9（C-20），34.2（C-21），33.2（C-22），28.8（C-23），15.5（C-24），16.6（C-25），17.4（C-26），26.2（C-27），180.2（C-28），33.3（C-29），23.7（C-30）

七、思考题

1. 用乙醇提取前先用水加热提取女贞子有什么作用？该操作否会损失齐墩果酸？

2. 在提取过程中为什么要加酸酸化？

3. 齐墩果酸还存在于哪些植物中？

4. 提取和分离齐墩果酸的方法还有哪些？

扫码"练一练"

Experiment ⅩⅤ Extraction, Isolation and Identification of Oleanolic Acid

1. Introductions

Oleanolic acid belonging to pentacyclic triterpene, has been found in many plants either in free state "aglycones" or in combined form as glycosides. The content of oleanolic acid could reach 8% in Fructus Ligustri Lucidi, which is the dried fruits of *Ligustrum lucidum* Ait. (Oleaceae family). The pharmacological investigation indicated that oleanolic acid could degrade transaminase and evidently protect hepatic injury induced by carbon tetrachloride. In clinical, it has been used mainly for therapy of acute icteric hepatitis, and it may ratherish contribute to chronic hepatitis.

2. Purposes

2. 1 Learn the extraction, isolation method of pentacyclic triterpene.

2. 2 Master the main properties of pentacyclic triterpene.

2. 3 Learn the utilization of TLC for the identification of pentacyclic triterpene such as oleanolic acid.

3. Principles

Oleanolic acid (3β-hydroxyolean-12-en-28-oic acid) are white needles in alcohol, m. p. 309 ~ 310℃, odorless, insipidity, MF $C_{30}H_{48}O_3$, MW 456. 71. It dissolves in methanol, alcohol, benzene, diethyl ethyl, acetone and chloroform, and it is insoluble in water.

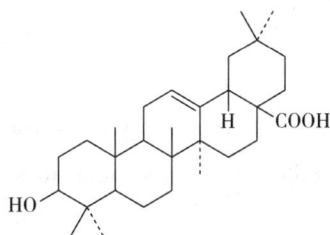

oleanolic acid

4. Apparatus and reagents

4. 1 Apparatus

Beaker (1000 ml), round-bottomed flask (250 ml), cylinder (100 ml), conical flask (500 ml), Büchner funnel, suction flask, condenser, vacuum pump, still head, adapter tube, Büchner filter, developing tank, microcapillary (1 mm), electric stove, baking oven, thermostat-controlled water bath, spraying bottle.

4. 2 Reagents

95% alcohol water solution, 6mol/L HCl, filter paper (5 cm × 8 cm), silica gel TLC.

5. Developing solvents and references

5. 1 Developing solvents

Petroleum-EtOAc (1 ∶ 1) (add a drop of acetic acid), cyclohexane-EtOAc (8 ∶ 2).

5. 2 Chromogenic agents

Vanillin-concentrated sulfate acid solution

5. 3 References

Oleanolic acid

6. Procedures

6. 1 Isolation and purification of oleanolic acid

6. 1. 1 Extraction and isolation

Weight Ligustri Lucidi Fructus (Nvzhenzi) 50 g, transfer itinto 1000 ml flask, add 300 ml water, soak for 4 days. Pour the infusion, add 300 ml water, heat to make the mixture boiled gently for 20 minutes, then pour the pulpy soup and abandon the testas and kernal separated from Nuzhenzi. Put fruit coats and pulp into the barking oven, dry them at 80 ~ 90℃, shatter, extract them with 50 ml 95% alcohol (10 times), reflux for 30 min twice. Combine two extracting solution, concentrate until half-volume solution. Add 1 ∶ 1 (volume ratio) water into concentrated solution, adjust pH to 1 with 6 mol/L HCl, keep the solution over night. Filter to get the precipitation. Dry, weight and calculate the yield.

6. 1. 2 Recrystallization

Dissolve 1 g of crude oleanolic acid with 90% ethanol as more as possible. Filter the hot solution to remove insoluble impurities, keep the solution to cool and deposit crystals of oleanolic acid. Filter the cold solution to afford purified oleanolic acid. Dry, weight and calculate the yield.

Alternative method: Dissolve 1 g of crude oleanolic acid with cyclohexane-EtOH (1 ∶ 1) as more as possible. Filter the solution to remove insoluble impurities. Allow the solution to cool and deposit crystals of oleanolic acid. Filter the cold solution to afford purified oleanolic acid. Dry, weight and calculate the yield.

6. 2 Identification

6. 2. 1 Color reaction

Put a few oleanolic acid into test tube, add 1 ml acetic anhydride, add a bit of drops of sulfuric acid along test tube wall. Between the juncture of two liquid layer, prunosus color cycle was observed.

6. 2. 2 TLC identification

Thin layer plate: silica gel G thin layer chromatography plate.

Samples: purified oleanolic acid, dissolved in 95% alcohol.

References: oleanolic acid, dissolved in 95% alcohol.

Developing solvents: Petroleum-EtOAc (3 ∶ 1) (add a drop of acetic acid), or cyclohexane-EtOAc (8 ∶ 2).

Imbibe appropriate amount of sample and reference solution with microcapillary, spot on the silica gel thin layer plate, develop by above developing solvents. After the developing solvent has volatilized, spray vanilline-concertrated sulfuric acid solution, heat it in the baking oven at 105℃ for 5 min. Oleanolic acid showed prunosus spot.

6. 2. 3 Identification by Spectral Data (See them in Chinese part.)

7. Questions

7. 1 Before extraction with EtOH, why hot water was applied to extract Nvzhenzi? Whether the content of oleanolic acid will be lost?

7. 2 During the extraction, why HCl was applied?

7. 3 Which plants are rich in oleanolic acid except for Nvzhenzi?

7. 4 What are the other extraction and isolation methods of oleanolic acid?

实验十六 薯蓣皂苷元的提取、分离和鉴定

一、简介

薯蓣皂苷元（diosgenin）是一种甾体皂苷元，在植物界主要分布在薯蓣科薯蓣属（dioscorea）植物中。我国的薯蓣属植物有 80 种，其中只有薯蓣根茎组（stenophora）的 17 种、1 亚种及 1 变种才含有甾体苷元，其他则含有大量淀粉，无皂苷元。已用于生产的主要有盾叶薯蓣（*Dioscorea zingiberensis* C. H. Wright）、穿龙薯蓣（*D. nipponica* Makino）、黄山药（*D. panthaica* Prain et Burk.）、黄独（*D. bulbifera* L）等。

20 世纪 30 年代中期，薯蓣皂苷元就已成为合成甾体激素类药物的重要原料，开创了利用植物原料进行甾体药物合成的先例。目前各国甾体激素类药物和甾体避孕药 60% 以上以薯蓣皂苷元为原料。穿山龙为薯蓣科植物穿龙薯蓣的干燥根茎，收于《中国药典》，是薯蓣皂苷元的重要药源之一。由于穿龙薯蓣具有薯蓣皂苷元含量高（约 1.5% ~ 2.6%）、易于栽培等特点而成为薯蓣皂苷元生产的重要原料来源。

二、目的

1. 掌握甾体皂苷元的提取方法。
2. 掌握甾体化合物的检识方法。
3. 掌握索氏提取器的应用。

三、原理

薯蓣皂苷元是一种甾体皂苷元，分子式为 $C_{27}H_{42}O_3$，分子量为 414.61，为白色结晶，熔点为 204 ~ 207℃，$[\alpha]_D^{25}$ – 129.3 °（$CHCl_3$），溶于一般有机溶剂和乙酸，不溶于水。在植物体内薯蓣皂苷元是与葡萄糖、鼠李糖结合成薯蓣皂苷（dioscin）而存在。提取分离时，一般是先用稀酸将薯蓣皂苷水解成薯蓣皂苷元与单糖（葡萄糖、鼠李糖），因薯蓣皂苷元不溶于水，混存于植物残渣中，故可用有机溶剂（如石油醚）直接从植物残渣中提取出薯蓣皂苷元。

扫码"学一学"

115

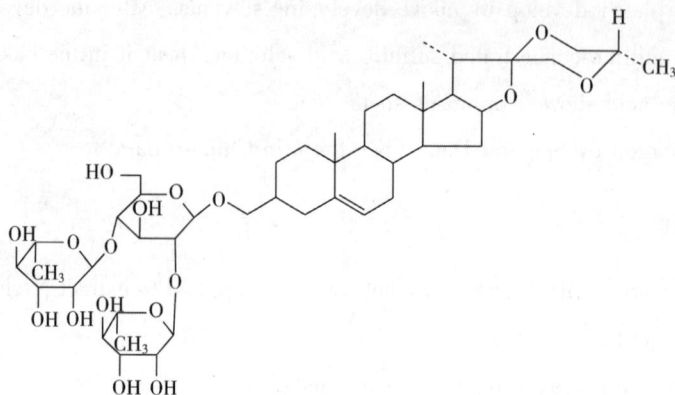

薯蓣皂苷元

四、仪器与试剂

1. **仪器** 圆底烧瓶（500 ml），三角烧瓶（500 ml×2，50 ml×5），玻璃漏斗（10 cm×2.5 cm），冷凝管（2 只），布氏漏斗＋抽滤瓶（500 ml），研钵，索氏提取器，滴管（3 只），试管（15 ml），蒸发皿，量筒（500 ml、50 ml、10 ml），水浴锅，循环水泵，电吹风，铁架台＋铁夹＋铁圈（2 套），电炉，石棉网，展开缸，点样毛细管（1mm）。

2. **试剂** 95% 乙醇，石油醚（60～90℃），醋酐，吡啶，丙酮，三氯醋酸，浓硫酸，碳酸钠，活性炭，硅胶 CMC－Na 板，滤纸，pH 试纸。

五、展开剂及对照品

1. **展开剂** 石油醚：乙酸乙酯（7∶3）。
2. **对照品** 薯蓣皂苷元。

六、操作

1. **薯蓣皂苷元的提取和纯化** 取穿山龙粗粉25g（过40目筛），置500ml 圆底烧瓶中，加8%酸水（水∶浓硫酸＝230∶20，V/V）250ml，然后直火加热（石棉网上），回流3.5h（开始时用小火，防止泡沫冲出）倒去酸水，加入常水洗涤2次，然后将药渣倒入研钵内，加固体碳酸钠粉研磨，调 pH 至中性，常水洗，过滤，滤渣研碎，低温干燥（不超过80℃）。将该干燥滤渣装入滤纸筒后置索氏提取器中，用石油醚（沸程60～90℃）300ml，在水浴上回流提取3h。提取液经常压回收石油醚至约10～15ml 时停止，用滴管将浓缩液转移入50ml 锥形瓶中，冷却，析出结晶，抽滤，用少量新鲜石油醚洗涤二次，即得薯蓣皂苷元粗品。粗品用20～30ml 95%乙醇加热溶解（色深时可加1%～2% 活性炭脱色），抽滤，滤液放置，析出结晶。滤出结晶，烘干，称重，计算得率。

2. **薯蓣皂苷元乙酰化物的制备** 取样品100mg溶于3ml 吡啶中，加入20ml 醋酐，煮沸半0.5～1.0 h 后，将反应物倒入冰水中（冬季操作使用冷水即可）。静置20min，待析出白色晶体后，抽滤，析出物丙酮重结晶即得。m. p. 为193～196℃。

3. **薯蓣皂苷元的检识**

（1）三氯醋酸反应（Rosen-Heimer reaction） 取薯蓣皂苷元结晶少许置于干燥试管中，加同量固体三氯醋酸放在60～70℃ 恒温水浴中加热，数分钟后由红→紫色。

（2）硫酸－醋酐反应（Liebermann-Burchard reaction） 取薯蓣皂苷元结晶少许溶于冰醋酸，加浓硫酸－醋酐（1∶20）试剂，观察颜色由红→紫→蓝→绿→污绿，最后褪色。

（3）三氯甲烷－浓硫酸反应（Salkowski reaction） 取薯蓣皂苷元结晶少许溶于三氯甲烷，沿管壁滴加浓硫酸，三氯甲烷层显血红色或青色，浓硫酸层显绿色荧光。

4. 薯蓣皂苷元的硅胶薄层鉴定

薄层板：硅胶 G 薄层层析板

样品溶液：自制薯蓣皂苷元少量以适量乙醇加热（或超声）溶解

对照品溶液：薯蓣皂苷元标准品乙醇溶液

展开剂：石油醚∶乙酸乙酯（7∶3）

用毛细管各吸取样品和对照品溶液适量，点于硅胶 G 薄层层析板上，用上述展开剂展开。硅胶 G 薄层层析板吹干后，均匀喷以 15% 硫酸乙醇液，电吹风加热，斑点呈紫红色→灰褐色。

5. 薯蓣皂苷元的 HPLC 色谱鉴定

色谱柱：TOSOH TSKgel OSD－100V 柱（4.6mm×250mm，5 μm）

流动相：甲醇

波长：203 nm

流速：0.8 ml/min

柱温：25℃

薯蓣皂苷元对照品 5mg，精密称定，置于 10ml 容量瓶中，甲醇溶解定容，得浓度为 500 μg/ml 的对照品溶液。自制薯蓣皂苷元样品 5mg 同法制备样品溶液。对照品及样品浓缩过 0.45 μm 微孔滤膜，吸取 10 μl 滤液，注入高效液相色谱仪，采用上述色谱条件，记录色谱图。对照品及样品均在 9.886min 处出现色谱峰。

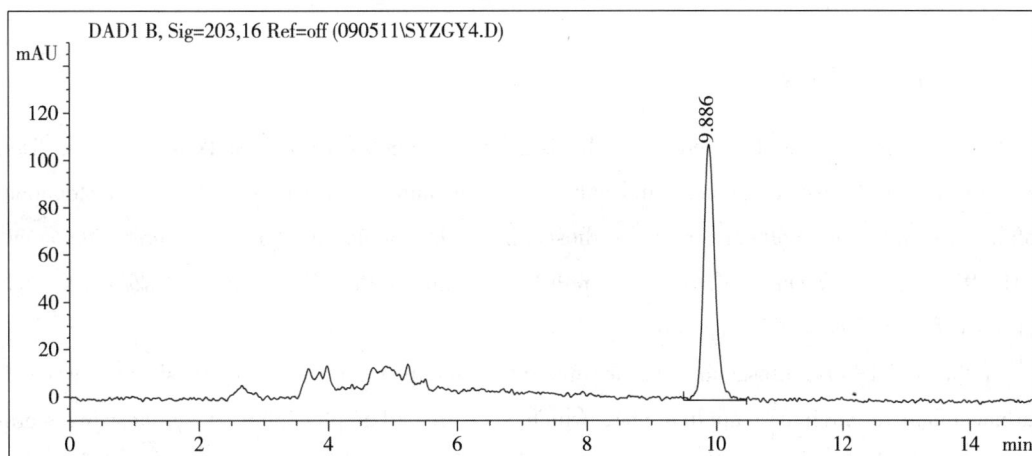

6. 光谱方法鉴别

UV（λ_{max}，nm）：203

IR（ν_{max}，KBr）：3451,3382（broad，OH），3028,2951,2929,2904,2872,2847,1456,1376,1303,1096,1053,1008920,899

EI-MS（m/z）：414（M）$^+$，139（100），282（41），300（25），271（20），69（17），55（16），41（15），115（15）

^{1}H-NMR（CDCl$_3$，600MHz）δ：5.36（1H，d，$J=3.6$ Hz，H-5），4.41（1H，dd，$J=10.0$，

5. 4 Hz, H-3）, 1. 03（3H, s, H-19）, 0. 97（3H, d, $J = 4.4$ Hz, H-21）, 0. 80（3H, s, H-18）, 0. 79（3H, d, $J = 4.4$ Hz, H-27）

^{13}C-NMR（CDCl$_3$, 150 MHz）δ：140. 8（C-5）, 121. 4（C-6）, 109. 3（C-22）, 80. 8（C-16）, 71. 7（C-3）, 66. 8（C-26）, 62. 1（C-17）, 56. 5（C-14）, 50. 1（C-9）, 42. 3（C-4）, 41. 6（C-20）, 40. 3（C-13）, 39. 8（C-12）, 37. 2（C-1）, 36. 6（C-10）, 32. 1（C-7）, 31. 8（C-15）, 31. 6（C-2）, 31. 44（C-8）, 31. 39（C-23）, 30. 3（C-25）, 28. 8（C-24）, 20. 9（C-11）, 19. 4（C-19）, 16. 3（C-18）, 14. 5（C-21）, 17. 1（C-27）

七、注意事项

1. 原料经酸水解后，应充分洗涤至中性，以免烘干时炭化。

2. 使用索氏提取器回流提取前，烧瓶内要加止爆剂。

3. 可用 Liebermann-Burchard 反应检查薯蓣皂苷元是否提取完全。

4. 索氏提取器为实验室中常用的提取仪器，通过溶剂蒸发、冷凝及仪器中的虹吸，使药渣中的物质每次经受纯净溶剂的溶解而被提取，效率极高，同时可节省溶剂。一般受热易分解或变色的物质或高沸点溶剂提取，本仪器不适用。

八、思考题

1. 重结晶操作应注意哪些问题？如何制成过饱和溶液？

2. 使用索氏提取器有什么优点，应注意哪些问题？

3. 三萜化合物和甾体类化合物在理化性质上有哪些不同之处，如何鉴别？

扫码"练一练"

Experiment XVI Extraction, Isolation and Identification of Diosgenin

1. Introductions

Diosgenin is a steroidal aglycon, which distribute in genus *Dioscorea* of Dioscoreaceae. There are more than 80 *Dioscorea* species, and only 17 species and 1 subspecies of the group Stenophora contain doisgenin, while others contain no diosgenin but lots of starch. Now, *Dioscorea zingiberensis* C. H. Wright, *D. nipponica* Makino, D. *panthaica* Prain et Burkill. , and *D. bulbifera* L. have been used for production of diosgenin.

In the mid-1930s, diosgenin was an important precursor for partial synthesis of steroids for pharmaceutical research and applications, which also created a precedent of synthesizing steroid hormones from plant material. At present, more than 60% steroid hormones and steroid contraceptive drugs are produced using diosgenin as raw material in every country. Dried root of *D. nipponica* Makino. , well known as Chuanshanlong, is one of the favorite traditional herbal medicine in China, and is officially listed in the *Chinese Pharmacopoeia*. Owing to the high contents of diosgenin and easy to cultivate, *D. nipponica* has become an important object of research.

2. Purposes

2. 1 Learn the extraction, isolation method of steroidal aglycon.

2.2 Familiar with the main properties of steroids.

2.3 Learn the utilization of Soxhlet extractor.

3. Principles

Diosgenin is white crystal, its molecular is $C_{27}H_{42}O_3$, the molecular weight 414.61, melting point is $204 \sim 207\,°C$, and the optical rotation value is $-129.3\,°(\,[\,\alpha\,]_D^{25}$, $CHCl_3\,)$. Diosgenin is soluble in common organic solvent and acetic acid, but insoluble in water. It often exists in plants as dioscin comprising one glucose and two rhamnose molecules linked to diosgenin. Because of its insolubility in water, diosgenin can be extracted from the plant residues by organic solvents, such as petroleum ether, after hydrolyzing dioscin to diosgenin and monosaccharides by dilute acid.

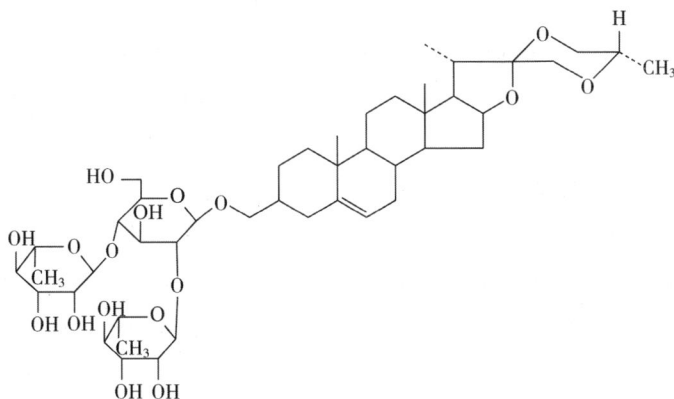

diosgenin

4. Apparatus and reagents

4.1 Apparatus

Flasks (500ml), conical flask (500 ml ×2, 50 ml ×5), glass funnel (10 cm ×2.5 cm), condenser, Büchner's filter + suction flask (500 ml), mortar, Soxhlet extractor, droppers (3 pieces), glass tubes (15 ml), evaporating basin, graduated flask (500 ml, 50 ml, 10 ml).

Thermostat-controlled water-bath, vacuum pump, electric hair-drier, iron stand + iron clip + iron ring (2 sets), electric stove, gauze with asbestos, developing chamber for TLC, glass sample capillary tube (1mm).

4.2 Reagents

95% ethanol, petroleum ether (60 ~ 90℃), acetic anhydride, pyridine, acetone, trichloro-acetic acid, concentrated sulfuric acid, Na_2CO_3, activated carbon, silica gel TLC plate, filter paper, pH test paper.

5. Developing solvents and references

5.1 Developing solvents

PE：EtOAc (7：3)

5.2 References

Diosgenin.

6. Procedures

6. 1 Isolation and purification of diosgenin

In a 500ml round bottom flask place 25g dry powder of Chuanshanlong, and 250ml of acid water (water : concentrated sulfuric acid = 230 : 20, V/V). Extract with direct fire on gauze with asbestos, reflux for 3. 5h, then remove acid water, wash the residues with water for 2 times. Pour the residues into mortar, grind with Na_2CO_3, adjust pH value to neutrality, wash with water then filter. Grind residues into fine power, dry with low temperature (not exceeding 80℃). Place the dry power in filtration paper cylinder, then put it into Soxhlet extractor, extract with 300ml petroleum ether (60~90 ℃) on a water bath for 3h. Concentrate extraction to 10 ~15 ml on water bath at normal pressure. Transfer the concentrate extraction into 50ml conical flask by dropper, cool the solution and precipitate crystals of diosgenin. Filter the cold solution to collect the crystals, recrystallize with 20 ~ 30ml 95% ethanol again to get purified diosgenin. Weigh and calculate the yield.

6. 2 Preparation of acetyl derivation

Dissolve 100mg diosgenin in 3ml pyridine, and 20ml acetic anhydride. Boil reaction solution 30minutes to 1h, pour it into ice water to deposit crystals. Let stand for 20 minutes to precipitate crystals, then filter to collect the crystals, recrystallize with acetone to get acetylate with m. p. 193~196℃.

6. 3 Examination of steroids

6. 3. 1 Rosen-heimer reaction

Put appropriate amount of diosgenin into a driedtube, add the same weight of solid trichloro-acrtic acid, heat on water bath at constant temperature 60~70℃. After several minutes, the color of the solvent changes from red to purple.

6. 3. 2 Liebermann-burchard reaction

Dissolve appropriate amount of diosgenin in glacial acetic acid, add the reagent of concentrated sulfuric acid-acetic anhydride (1 : 20), observe that the color of the solvent changes from red to purple, then to blue and green, and fade finally.

6. 3. 3 Salkowski reaction

Dissolve appropriate amount of diosgenin in chloroform, drop concentrated sulfuric acid along tube wall, the color of chloroform layer show sanguine or cerulean green while sulfuric acid layer green fluorescence.

6. 4 Identification of diosgenin

TLC plate: Silica gel CMC-Na plate.

Sample: Prepared diosgenin, dissolved in ethanol.

Reference: Diosgenin for reference, dissolved in ethanol.

Developing Solvent: PE : EtOAc (7 : 3).

Appropriate amount of sample and reference solutions werespotted with glass capillary tube, developed by the above developing solvent. Sprinkle 15% sulphuric acid ethanol solution, heat plate by electric hair-drier, the spots show purplish red to beige color.

6. 5 HPLC chromatography

Chromatography column: TOSON TSKgel OSD – 100V column (4. 6mm × 250mm, 5μm).

Mobile phase: Methanol.

Detection wavelength: 203nm.

Flow rate: 0. 8ml/min.

Column temperature: 25℃.

Accurately weight 5mg reference and sample, then dissolve in methanol to get stock solution of 500 μg/ml respectively. The obtained solutions are filtered through a syringe filter (0. 45μm), 10μl aliquots were subjected to HPLC, and determined by the proposed HPLC-UV at the conditions above. Record the chromatograms, show chromatographic peaks of reference and sample at 9. 886 min respectively.

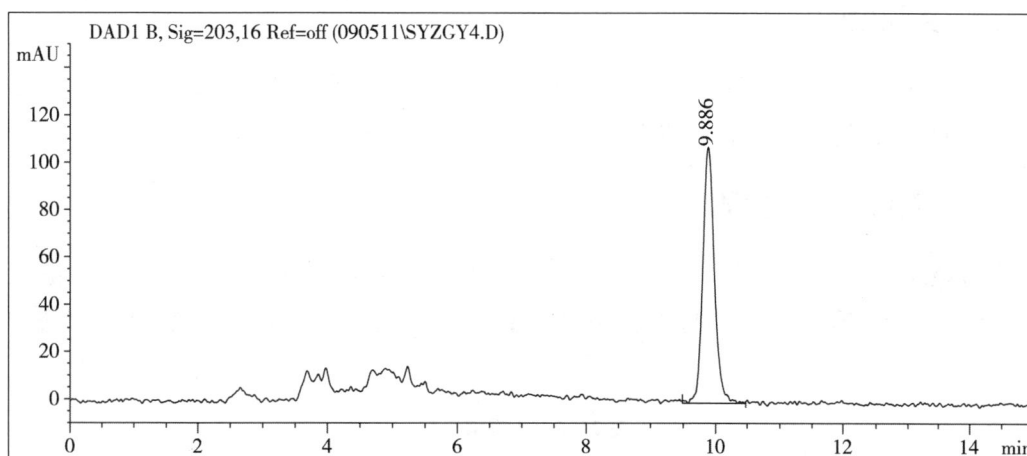

6. 6 Identified by spectral data (See them in Chinese part.)

7. Notices

7. 1 Wash the raw material to neutrality to avoid carbonization when drying, after hydrolyzed by acid.

7. 2 Before reflux with Soxhlet extractor, add the antidetonator into flasks.

7. 3 Use Liebermann-Burchard reaction to check whether diosgenin is already extracted completely.

7. 4 Soxhlet's extractor is the most common extract apparatus in the laboratories. By solvents vaporixation, condensation, and siphon, the compounds in raw material are extracted effectively by dissolving with clean solvents, which can save solvents. This apparatus is not suitable for extraction of easily degradable material or solvents with high boiling points.

8. Questions

8. 1 What should be paid attention to, when do the operation of recrystallization? How can you make supersaturated solvents?

8. 2 What are the advantages of using Soxhlet apparatus? What kind of points should be paid attention to?

8.3 What physicochemical properties are different between triterpene and steroid? How can you identify them?

实验十七　天然产物化学成分系统预实验

一、简介

天然产物中含有多种化学成分，在深入研究之前应首先了解其中有哪些类型的化学成分。利用各类成分的颜色反应和沉淀反应，对天然产物的提取液进行检查可以初步判断其中的化学成分。由于提取液的颜色通常较深，影响对颜色变化的观察，可以使用薄层色谱（TLC）或纸色谱（PC）等方法对天然产物的提取液进行初步分离，再进一步检查。

二、实验目的

掌握未知成分的天然产物是怎样初步提取分离，熟悉各主要成分的试管试验、沉淀反应和纸色谱、薄层色谱的方法并根据试验结果判断所含化学成分类型。

三、实验方法及过程

1. **水浸液**　取 5 g 中药粉末加 60 ml 水，在 50~60℃的水浴上加热 1h 后过滤，滤液做表 2-6 试验。（有 * 标记的在试管中进行；有 # 标记的在滤纸或硅胶薄层板上进行，下同。）

表 2-6　水提液试验

检查项目	试剂及方法	现象	结论
糖	*酚醛缩合反应：试液于试管内加 α-萘酚试剂 1~2 滴，振摇后倾斜试管，沿试管壁加浓硫酸几滴，观察在两液接触面变化		
	*菲林反应：将甲乙液各滴 3 滴至试管混匀后加试液，看现象		
有机酸	# pH 试纸检查		
	# 溴甲酚绿试剂检查：试液点于滤纸上，喷溴甲酚绿试剂		
酚类、鞣质	#1% 三氯化铁试剂：显蓝、墨绿或蓝紫色		
	*明胶试剂：有沉淀产生		
氨基酸	#茚三酮试剂：点试液及茚三酮于试纸上，110℃烤 2 min		
蛋白质	*双缩脲反应：取甲乙液等量混合后，加入 1ml 试液震摇，冷却观察现象		
苷类和多糖	*酚醛缩合反应		
	*加 6 mol/L 盐酸酸化煮沸数分钟，冷却，观察有无沉淀		
	*菲林试剂：观察水解前后氧化亚铜沉淀有无增加		
皂苷	*泡沫实验：1ml 试液震摇 1min，放置 10min，观察泡沫是否消失		
生物碱	*碘化铋钾试剂		
	*硅钨酸试剂		

2. **乙醇提取液**　取中药粉末适量，加 5~12 倍量的工业酒精，在水浴锅上回流提取 1h，过滤，滤液留 3ml 做表 2-7 各项实验。其余滤液回收乙醇至无醇味，并浓缩成浸膏状

（注意不要蒸干），分成两份，一份加少量2%的盐酸溶解，过滤。滤液做表2-8中各项实验；滤饼用乙醇溶解后做表2-9中各项检查。

另一份浸膏用少量乙酸乙酯溶解，溶液置分液漏斗中加适量5%氢氧化钠震摇，使酚性物质及有机酸等转入下层碱溶液中，乙酸乙酯层为中性化合物部分。分取乙酸乙酯层，用蒸馏水洗至中性，取乙酸乙酯液3~5ml于蒸发皿中，水浴蒸干，以2~4ml乙醇溶解做表2-10中各项检查。

表2-7　醇提液试验①

检查项目	试剂	现象	结论
酚类	#1%三氯化铁试剂		
鞣质			
有机酸	溴甲酚绿试剂		

表2-8　醇提液试验②

检查项目	试剂	现象	结论
生物碱	*碘化铋钾试剂		
	*硅钨酸试剂		
	*鞣酸试剂		
	*苦味酸试剂		

表2-9　醇提液试验③

检查项目	试剂及方法	现象	结论
黄酮	#1%三氯化铝试剂：黄色斑点；紫外灯下		
	*盐酸镁粉反应：取试液水浴加热加盐酸2滴后加少量镁粉，观察溶液变化		
蒽醌	#10%KOH液		
	#醋酸镁试剂		
	#氨熏		

表2-10　醇提液试验④

检查项目	试剂及方法	现象	结论
香豆素与萜类内酯	*开闭环反应：取1ml试液加2ml 1%氢氧化钠，沸水浴3分钟。观察液体在加入2%盐酸前后变化		
	#氨基安替比林-铁氰化钾显色反应：将试液点于滤纸上先喷Ⅰ再喷Ⅱ即显色		
	*羟胺反应：取1ml试液加新鲜的甲液0.5ml，加2N氢氧化钾0.5ml使溶液呈碱性，水浴微热，冷却后加1%三氯化铁的盐酸溶液1~2滴后滴加5%盐酸使溶液呈微酸性，观察现象		
强心苷	# Kedde试剂		
	*苦味酸试剂：滴加后静止一刻钟，观察色泽变化，注意空白对照		

3. 石油醚提取液 取中药粉末1g，加10ml石油醚，放置2~3小时，过滤，置表面皿上任其挥发，用残留物进行表2-11中实验。

表2-11 石油醚提取液试验

检查项目	试剂及方法	现象	结论
甾体或三萜类	*醋酐浓硫酸实验：观察颜色变化		
	# 磷钼酸试剂		
挥发油和油脂	石油醚提取液滴于滤纸上，观察有无油斑并观察其加热后能否挥发		

综合以上六个表格的实验现象，编号为_____的药材中：

一定含有的化学成分类型：

可能含有的化学成分类型：

不含有的化学成分类型：

实验报告人 学号_____，姓名_____

学号_____，姓名_____

四、主要试剂及配制方法

1. 生物碱沉淀试剂

（1）碘化铋钾（Dragendorff）试剂 取次硝铋钾8g溶于30%硝酸（比重1.18）17ml中，在搅拌下慢慢加碘化钾浓水溶液（27g碘化钾溶于20ml水），静置1夜，取上层清液，加蒸馏水稀释至100ml。

（2）碘化汞钾（Mayer）试剂 氯化汞1.36g和碘化钾5g各溶于20ml水中，混合后加水稀释至100ml。

（3）碘-碘化钾（Wagner）试剂 1g碘和10g碘化钾溶于50ml水中，加热，加2ml醋酸，再用水稀释至100ml。

（4）硅钨酸试剂 5g硅钨酸溶于100ml水中，加盐酸少量至pH 2左右。

（5）苦味酸试剂 1g苦味酸溶于100ml水中。

（6）鞣酸试剂 鞣酸1g加乙醇1ml溶解后再加水至10ml。

（7）硫酸铈-硫酸试剂 0.1g硫酸铈混悬于4ml水中，加入1g三氯醋酸，加热至沸，逐滴加入浓硫酸至澄清。

2. 苷类检出试剂

（1）糖的检出试剂

①碱性酒石酸铜（Fehling）试剂 本品分甲液与乙液，应用时等量混合。

甲液：结晶硫酸铜 6.23g，加水至 100ml。

乙液：酒石酸钾钠 34.6g，及氢氧化钠 10g，加水至 100ml。

②α-萘酚（Molisch）试剂

甲液：α-萘酚 1g，加 75% 乙醇至 10ml。

乙液：浓硫酸

③氨性硝酸银试剂　硝酸银 1g，加水 20ml 溶解，注意滴加适量的氨水，随加随拌，至开始产生的沉淀将近全溶为止，过滤。

（2）α-去氧糖显色试剂

①三氯化铁冰醋酸（Keller-Killiani）试剂

甲液：1% 三氯化铁溶液 0.5ml，加冰醋酸至 100ml。

乙液：浓硫酸

②呫吨氢醇冰醋酸（Xanthydrol）试剂　呫吨氢醇溶于 100ml 冰醋酸（含 1% 的盐酸）中

3. 酚类检出试剂

（1）三氯化铁试剂　5% 三氯化铁的水溶液或醇溶液。

（2）三氯化铁 – 铁氰化钾试剂　应用时甲液、乙液等体积混合。

甲液：三氯化铁 2g 溶于 100ml 水中。

乙液：铁氰化钾 1g 溶于 100ml 水中。

（3）4 – 氨基安替比林 – 铁氰化钾（Emersen）试剂

甲液：4 – 氨基安替比林 2g 溶于 100ml 乙醇中。

乙液：铁氰化钾 8g 溶于 100ml 水中。

（4）重氮化试剂

甲液：对硝基苯胺 0.35g，溶于浓盐酸 5ml 中，加水至 50ml。

乙液：亚硝酸钠 5g，加水至 50ml。

应用时取甲、乙液等量在冰水浴中混合后，方可使用。

（本试剂宜临用时配制）

（5）Gibb's 试剂

甲液：2，6 – 二氯苯醌氯亚胺 0.5g 溶于 100ml 的乙醇中。

乙液：硼酸 – 氯化钾 – 氢氧化钾缓冲液（pH9.4）。

4. 内酯、香豆素类检出试剂

（1）羟胺试剂

甲液：新鲜配制的 1mol/L 羟胺盐酸盐（M = 69.5）的甲醇液。

乙液：1.1mol/L 氢氧化钾（M = 56.1）的甲醇液。

丙液：三氯化铁溶于 1% 的盐酸溶液。

甲、乙液混合后再加丙液。

（2）4 – 氨基安替比林 – 铁氰化钾（Emersen）试剂

（3）重氮化试剂

（4）开环 – 闭环试剂

甲液：1% 氢氧化钠溶液。

乙液：2% 盐酸溶液。

5. 黄酮类检出试剂

（1）盐酸镁粉试剂　浓盐酸和镁粉。

（2）三氯化铝试剂　三氯化铝 2g 溶于 100ml 甲醇中。

（3）醋酸镁试剂　醋酸镁 1g 溶于 100ml 甲醇中。

（4）碱式醋酸铅试剂　取一氧化铅 14g，加水 10ml，研磨成糊状，用水 10ml 洗入玻璃瓶中。加醋酸铅 22g 的水溶液 70ml，用力振摇 5min 后，时时振摇。放置 7 天，过滤，加新沸过的冷水至 100ml。

6. 蒽醌类检出试剂

（1）氢氧化钾试剂　氢氧化钾 10g 溶于 100ml 水中。

（2）醋酸镁试剂　醋酸镁 10g 溶于 100ml 甲醇中。

（3）1% 硼酸试剂　硼酸 1g 溶于 100ml 水中。

（4）浓硫酸试剂　浓硫酸。

（5）碱式醋酸铅试剂。

7. 强心苷类检出试剂

（1）3，5 – 二硝基苯甲酸（Kedde）试剂

甲液：2%3，5 – 二硝基苯甲酸甲醇液。

乙液：1mol/L 氢氧化钾甲醇溶液。

应用前甲、乙两液等量混合。

（2）碱性苦味酸（Baljet）试剂

甲液：1% 苦味酸水溶液。

乙液：10% 氢氧化钠溶液。

（3）亚硝基铁氰化钠 – 氢氧化钠（Legal）试剂

甲液：吡啶。

乙液：0.5% 亚硝基铁氰化钠溶液。

丙液：10% 氢氧化钠溶液。

8. 皂苷类检出试剂

（1）醋酐 – 浓硫酸（Liebermann – Berchard）试剂

甲液：醋酐。

乙液：浓硫酸。

（2）浓硫酸试剂　浓硫酸。

（3）氰苷类　苦味酸钠试剂：适当大小的滤纸条，浸入苦味酸的饱和水溶液，浸透后取出晾干，再浸入 10% 碳酸钠水溶液中，迅速取出晾干即得。

9. 萜类、甾体类检出试剂

（1）香草醛 – 浓硫酸试剂　0.5g 香草醛溶于 100ml 硫酸 – 乙醇（4：1）中。

（2）三氯化锑（Carr – price）试剂　25g 三氯化锑溶于 75g 三氯甲烷中。

（3）间二硝基苯试剂　甲液：2% 间二硝基苯乙醇液。

乙液：14% 氢氧化钾甲醇液。

用前甲、乙两液等量混合。

10. 鞣质类检出试剂

（1）三氯化铁试剂　5g 三氯化铁溶于水或乙醇中制成 100ml 溶液。

（2）三氯化铁 – 铁氰化钾试剂。

（3）4 – 氨基安替比林 – 铁氰化钾试剂

甲液：2g 4 – 氨基安体比林溶于 100ml 乙醇中。

乙液：8g 铁氰化钾溶于 100ml 乙醇中。

（4）明胶试剂　10g 氯化钠，1g 明胶，加水至 100ml。

11. 氨基酸多肽、蛋白质检出试剂

（1）双缩脲（Biuret）试剂

甲液：1％硫酸铜溶液。

乙液：40％氢氧化钠液。

应用前甲乙两液等量混合。

（2）茚三酮试剂　0.2g 茚三酮溶于 100 ml 乙醇。

（3）鞣酸试剂。

12. 有机酸检出试剂　溴麝香草酚蓝试剂：0.1g 溴麝香草酚蓝溶于 100ml 乙醇液。

五、练习

根据实验结果，写出样品中所含的化学成分类型。

Experment ⅩⅦ　The Systemic Preparative Test on Chemical Components of Nature Products

1. Introduction

There are many kinds of categories ingredients in nature products. We should know what kinds of components in it before thoroughly study. Components can be primary estimated depending on the result of color test and precipitation reaction with extract. Owing to the color of the extract is usually too deep to be observed, we could separate it by means of thin layer chromatography and paper chromatography before test.

2. Purpose

From this experiment, students will learn how to extract unknown nature products, know the color test or precipitation reaction of the main constituents, comprehend the method of TLC and PC, and estimate the categories of constituents depending on the results.

3. Procedures

Depending on the solubility of different constituents is various in different solvent, we can extract the sample by three kind of solvents respectively and test them by following reagents.

3. 1 Water extract

Place some of coarse sample powder in water, heat at $50^{\circ}\text{C} \sim 60^{\circ}\text{C}$ on a water bath for an

扫码"练一练"

hour， filter， test the filtrate by different test solution（table 2 – 6）．

Table 2 – 6. test for constituents from water extract

Check item	Reagents and methods	Phenomenon	Conclusion
sugar	＊ Phenolic condensation reaction： add 1 or 2 drops of α-naphthol reagent to the test solution. Tilt the test tube after shaking, add a few drops of concentrated sulfuric acid along the test tube wall, and generate a reddish-red ring on the contact surface of the two liquids.		
	＊ Fehling's solution： add 3 drops of A and B liquid to the test tube, add the test solution, and see the phenomenon		
organic acid	# pH test paper check		
	# Bromocresol green reagent inspection： the test solution is spotted on the filter paper, and the bromocresol green reagent is sprayed		
phenols, tannins	# 1% Ferric chloride reagent： blue, dark green, or blue-violet		
	＊ Gelatin reagent： precipitation occurs		
amino acid	# Ninhydrin reagent： spot test solution and ninhydrin on the test paper, bake for 2 minutes at 110 ℃		
protein	＊ Biuret reaction： after mixing equal amounts of methyl ethyl solution, add 1mL of test solution to shake, and see the phenomenon		
glycosides and polysaccharides	＊ Phenolic condensation reaction		
	＊ Add 6mol/L hydrochloric acid to boil for several minutes, cool, and observe whether there is precipitation		
	＊ Fehling's solution: observe whether the precipitation of cuprous oxide increases before and after hydrolysis		
saponin	＊ Foam experiment: shake 1ml of test solution for 1 minute, leave it for 10 minutes, and observe whether the foam disappears		
alkaloid	＊ Bismuth potassium iodide reagent： orange red or yellow precipitation		
	＊ Silotungstic acid reagent： light yellow or off-white precipitate appears		

＊ Test in tube, #Test on PC or TLC-CMC-Na（the same below）

3. 2 Ethanol extract

Place some of coarse sample powder in 5 ~ 12 times amounts of 95% ethanol, heated under reflux for an hour, filter. To 3ml of filtrate use for test① （table 2 –7）, others condensed to extract. Divided the extract into two parts, one of them dissolved in a little 2% HCl, filter, seperate the acid solution for test② （table 2 – 8）, dissolve the residue on the filter paper in ethanol for test ③ （table 2 –9）．

Dissolve the other part of extract in a little ethyl acetate, transfer the solution to a separatory funnel, add appropriate amount of 5% NaOH, shake well. Phenolics and organic acid were dissolved in the under layer, neutral constituents remain in up layer. Wash ethyl acetate with water to neutral, evaporate 3 ~ 5ml on a water bath, dissolve the residue in 2 ~ 4ml ethanol for test④ （table 2 – 10）．

Table 2 – 7. test for constituents from ethand extract ①

Check item	Reagents	Phenomenon	Conclusion
Phenols	# 1% Ferric chloride reagent		
Tannins			
Organic acid	* Bromocresol green reagent		

Table 2 – 8. test for constituents from ethand extract②

Check item	Reagents	Phenomenon	Conclusion
Alkaloid	* Bismuth potassium iodide reagent		
	* Silicon Tungstic Acid Reagent		
	* Tannin reagent		
	* Picric acid reagent		

Table 2 – 9. test for constituents from ethand extract③

Check item	Reagents and methods	phenomenon	conclusion
Flavone	# 1% Aluminum trichloride reagent; yellow spots		
	* Magnesium hydrochloride powder reaction: take the test solution in a water bath and add 2 drops of hydrochloric acid, then add a small amount of magnesium powder. The solution changes from yellow to red to be a positive reaction.		
Anthraquinone	# 10% KOH solution		
	#Magnesium acetate reagent		
	# Ammonia smoke		

Table 2 – 10. test for constituents from ethand extract④

Check item	Reagents and methods	phenomenon	conclusion
Coumarin and terpenoids	* Open-closed loop reaction: Take 1ml test solution, add 2ml 1% sodium hydroxide, and bath in boiling water for 3 minutes. See the phenomenon of liquid before and after adding 2% hydrochloric acid		
	#Amino antipyrine-potassium ferricyanide color reaction: point the test solution on the filter paper first spray I and then spray II to develop color		
	* Hydroxyamine reaction: Take 1ml of test solution, add 0.5ml of fresh nail solution, add 2N potassium hydroxide 0.5ml to make the solution alkaline, heat slightly in the water bath, add 1 to 2 drops of 1% ferric chloride hydrochloric acid solution after cooling Add 5% hydrochloric acid dropwise to make the solution slightly acidic and see the phenomenon		
Cardioside	#Kedde reagent		
	* Picric acid reagent: stand for a quarter of an hour after the addition, see the phenmenon and pay attention to the blank control.		

(3) Petroleum ether extract

Place 1g of coarse sample powder in 10ml petroleum ether (boiling range 60~90℃), allow to stand for 2~3 hours, filter. Place the filtate in an evaporating dish, allow it to evaporate, the residue used as following test (table 2 – 11).

Table 2 – 11. test for constituents from petroleum ether extract

Check item	Reagents and methods	phenomenon	conclusion
Steroids or Triterpenes	∗ Acetic anhydrideconcentrated sulfuric acid experiment: observe the change of the color		
	#Phosphomolybdic acid reagent		
Essential oils and greases	Drops of petroleum ether extract on the filter paper, observe whether there are oil spots and observe whether it can volatilize after heating		

4. Main Reagents and Preparing

4. 1 Test solution for Alkaloids

4. 1. 1 Potassium iodobismuthate reagent

Place 8g of iodobismuthate in 17ml of 30% nitric acid (specific gravity1. 18), add potassium iodine water solution (dissolve 27g of potassium iodine in 20ml water) slowly with stirring. Allow to stand for a night, separate clear layer, dilute with water to 100ml.

4. 1. 2 Mayer reagent

Dissolve 1. 36g mercuric chloride and 5g potassium iodine in 20ml water, mix well and dilute with water to 100ml.

4. 1. 3 Wagner reagent

Dissolve 1g iodine and 10g potassium iodine in 50ml of water, heat and add 2ml acetic acid, dilute with water to 100ml.

4. 1. 4 Silicowolframic acid reagent

Dissolve 5g Silicowolframic acid in 100ml water, adjust the pH value to 2 with a little hydrochloric acid.

4. 1. 5 Trinitrophenol reagent

Dissolve 1g trinitrophenol in water to produce 100ml.

4. 1. 6 Tannic acid reagent

Dissolve 1g tannic acid in water, add 1ml ethanol and sufficient water to make 100ml.

4. 1. 7 Ceric sulfate-sulfuric acid reagent

Place 0. 1g ceric sulfate in 4ml of water, add 1g of trichloroacetic acid, heat to boiled, add sulfuric acid dropwise to completely clear.

4. 2 Test solution for glycosides

4. 2. 1 Reagents for sugar

4. 2. 1. 1 Fehling reagents

(ii) Dissolve 6. 23g cupric sulfate in water to make 100ml.

(iii) Place 34. 6g potassium tartrate and 10g of sodium hydroxide in water to produce 100ml.

Mix equal parts of the two solutions immediately before use.

4. 2. 1. 2 Molisch reagent

（ⅰ）Place 1gα-naphthol in 75% ethanol to make 10ml.

（ⅱ）Concentrated sulfuric acid

4. 2. 1. 3 Ammoniated silver nitrate Reagent

Dissolve 1g silver nitrate in 20ml of water，add ammonia Reagents dropwise with stirring until the precipitate is almost completely dissolved，filter.

4. 2. 2 Reagents for α-deoxysugar or α-dexyribose

4. 2. 2. 1 Keller-Killiani reagent

（ⅰ）Add 0. 5ml 1% ferric chloride in acetic acid glacial to produce 100ml.

（ⅱ）Concentrated sulfuric acid

4. 2. 2. 2 Xanthydrol reagent

Dissolve xanthydrol in 100ml of acetic acid glacial（contain 1% HCl）.

4. 3 Test solution for phenolics

4. 3. 1 Ferric chloride reagent

Dissolve 5g ferric chloride in water or ethanol to make 100ml.

4. 3. 2 Ferride chloride-potassium ferricyanide Reagent

（ⅰ）Dissolve 2g ferric chloride in water to make 100ml.

（ⅱ）Dissolve 1g potassium ferricyanide in water to make 100ml.

Mix equal parts of the two solutions immediately before use.

4. 3. 3 Emersen Reagent

（ⅰ）Dissolve 2g 4-amino-antipyrine in ethanol to make 100ml.

（ⅱ）Dissolve 8g potassium ferricyanide in water to make 100ml.

4. 3. 4 Diazotized ρ-Nitroaniline Reagents

（ⅰ）Dissolve 0. 35g ρ-Nitroaniline in 5ml concentrated hydrochloric acid，add water to make 50ml.

（ⅱ）Place 5g sodium nitrite in water to produce 50ml.

Mix equal parts of the two solutions in cool water immediately before use.（This solution must be freshly prepared）

4. 3. 5 Gibb's reagent

（ⅰ）Dissolve 0. 5g 2,6-dichloroquinone-chlorimide in 100ml of ethanol.

（ⅱ）Boric acid-potassium chloride-potassium hydroxide buffer solutions（pH9. 4）

4. 4 Test solution for lactone and coumarin

4. 4. 1 Hydroxylamine reagent

（ⅰ）Fresh prepared 1mol/L of hydroxylamine hydrochloride（M = 69. 5）methanol solution.

（ⅱ）1. 1mol/L potassium hydroxide（M = 56. 1）methanol solution.

（ⅲ）Dissolve ferric chloride in 1% hydrochloric acid.

Add the third solution after the first two solutions were mix well throughly.

4. 4. 2 Emersen reagent

4. 4. 3 Diazotized ρ-Nitroaniline reagent

4. 4. 4 Open and closed ring test solution

4. 4. 4. 1 1% sodium hydroxide solution.

4. 4. 4. 2 2% hydrochloric acid solution.

4. 5 Test solution for flavonoids

4. 5. 1 Hydrochloric acid-magnesium

Concentrated hydrochloric acid and magnesium.

4. 5. 2 Aluminium trichloride reagent

Dissolve 2g aluminium in methanol to produce 100ml.

4. 5. 3 Magnesium acetate reagent

Dissolve 1g magnesium acetate in methanol to produce 100ml.

4. 5. 4 Alkaline lead acetate reagent

Triturate 14g of lead monoxide with 10ml of water to make a paste, transfer to a glass bottle with 10ml of water, add a solution of 22g lead acetate in 70ml of water, shake vigorously for 5 minutes. Allow to stand for 7 days with occasional shaking, filter ang add fresh boiled and cooled water to produce 100ml.

4. 6 Test solution for anthraquinones

4. 6. 1 Potassium hydroxide reagent

Dissolve 10g potassium hydroxide in water to produce 100ml.

4. 6. 2 Magnesium acetate reagent

Dissolve 10g magnesium acetate in methanol to produce 100ml.

4. 6. 3 Boric acid reagents

Dissolve 1g boric acid in water to produce 100ml.

4. 6. 4 Sulfuric acid reagent

Concentrated sulfuric acid.

4. 6. 5 Alkaline lead acetate reagent

4. 7 Test solution for cardiac glycoside

4. 7. 1 Kedde reagent

4. 7. 1. 1 2% 3, 5-Dinitrobenzoic acid methanol solution.

4. 7. 1. 2 1mol/L potassium hydroxide methanol solution.

Mix equal parts of the two solutions immediately before use.

4. 7. 2 Baljet reagent

4. 7. 2. 1 1% trinitrophenol water solution.

4. 7. 2. 2 10% sodium hydroxide solution.

4. 7. 3 Legal reagent

4. 7. 3. 1 Pyridine

4. 7. 3. 2 0. 5% sodium nitroprusside solution.

4. 7. 3. 3 10% sodium hydroxide solution.

4. 8 Test solution for saponins

4. 8. 1 Liebermann-berchard reagent

4. 8. 1. 1 Acetic anhydride

4. 8. 1. 2 Concentrated sulfuric acid.

4. 8. 2 Sulfuric acid reagent

Concentrated sulfuric acid.

4.8.3 Cyanogenic glycoside

Sodium Trinitrophenol Reagent

Put a piece of appropriate size of filter paper in saturation trinitrophenol water solution and than into 10% sodium carbonate solution, take out at once and air the paper.

4.9 Test solution for terpenes and steroids

4.9.1 Vanillin-sulfuric acid reagent

Dissolve 0.5g boric acid in sulfuric acid-ethanol (4 : 1) to produce 100ml.

4.9.2 Carr-price Reagent

Dissolve 25g antimony trichloride in 75g $CHCl_3$.

4.9.3 *m*-dinitrobenzene reagent

（ⅰ） 2% *m*-dinitrobenzene ethanol solution.

（ⅱ） 14% potassium hydroxide methanol solution.

Mix equal parts of the two solutions immediately before use.

4.10 Test solution for tannins

4.10.1 Ferric chloride reagent

Dissolve 5g of ferric chloride in water or ethanol to make 100ml.

4.10.2 Ferride chloride-potassium ferricyanide Reagent

4.10.3 Emersen reagent

（ⅰ） Dissolve 2g of 4-amino-antipyrine in ethanol to make 100ml.

（ⅱ） Dissolve 8g of potassium ferricyanide in ethanol to make 100ml.

4.10.4 Gelatin reagent

Place 10g of sodium chloride and 1g of gelatin in water to produce 100ml.

4.11 Test solution for amino acid and protein

4.11.1 Biuret reagent

（ⅰ） 1% cupric sulfate solution.

（ⅱ） 40% sodium hydroxide solution.

Mix equal parts of the two solutions immediately before use.

4.11.2 Ninhydrin reagent

Dissolve 0.2g ninhydrin in ethanol to produce 100ml.

4.11.3 Tannic acid reagent

4.12 Test solution for organic acid

Bromothymol blue reagent

Dissolve 0.1g bromothymol blue in ethanol to produce 100ml.

5. Exersise

Write down the kinds of constituents in the sample depending on the result you have tested.

附　录

附录一　常用有机溶剂及有关数据表

溶剂的极性与洗脱能力大小决定于溶剂的分子结构，在很大程度上可以用解电常数来比较。

附表1　常用溶剂性质

溶剂名称及结构	沸点	解电常数	溶解度（20~25℃）	
			溶剂在水中	水在溶剂中
石油醚	30~60℃	1.80	不溶	不溶
正己烷 C_6H_{14}	69℃	1.88	0.00095%	0.0111%
环己烷	81℃	2.02	0.010%	0.0055%
二氧六环	101℃	2.21	任意	混溶
四氯化碳 CCl_4	77℃	2.24	0.077%	0.010%
苯	80℃	2.29	0.1780%	0.063%
甲苯	111℃	2.37	0.1515%	0.0334%
间二甲苯	137℃	2.38	0.0176%	0.5402%
二硫化碳 CS_2	46℃	2.34	0.294%	<0.005%
乙醚 $(C_2H_5)_2O$	35℃	4.34	6.04%	1.168%
醋酸戊酯 $CH_3COOC_5H_{11}$	149℃	4.75	0.17%	1.15%
三氯甲烷 $CHCl_3$	61℃	4.81	0.815%	0.072%
醋酸乙酯 $CH_3COOC_2H_5$	77℃	6.02	8.08%	2.94%
醋酸 CH_3COOH	118℃	6.15	任意	混溶
苯胺	184℃	6.89	3.38%	4.76%
苯酚	180℃	9.78（60℃）	8.66%	28.72%
1，1-二氯乙烷 CH_3CHCl_2	57℃	10	6.03%	<0.2%
1，2-二氯乙烷 CH_2ClCH_2Cl	84℃	10.4	0.81%	0.15%
吡啶	115℃	12.3	任意	混溶
叔丁醇 $(CH_3)_3COH$	82℃	12.47	任意	混溶
正戊醇 $n\text{-}C_5H_{11}OH$	138℃	13.9	2.19%	7.41%
异戊醇 $(CH_3)_2CH_2CH_2OH$	131℃	14.7	2.67%	9.61%
仲丁醇 $CH_3CHOHC_2H_5$	100℃	16.56	12.5%	44.1%
正丁醇 $n\text{-}C_4H_9OH$	118℃	17.8	7.45%	20.5%
环己酮	157℃	18.3	2.3%	8.0%
甲乙酮 $CH_3COC_2H_5$	80℃	18.5	24%	10.0%
异丙醇 $\begin{array}{c}CH_3\\\diagdown\\CHOH\\\diagup\\CH_3\end{array}$	82℃	19.92	任意	混溶

续表

溶剂名称及结构	沸点	解电常数	溶解度 (20～25℃)	
			溶剂在水中	水在溶剂中
正丙醇 n-C$_3$H$_7$OH	97℃	20.3	任意	混溶
酯酐 CH$_3$CO–O–CH$_3$CO	140℃	20.7	微溶	微溶
丙酮 CH$_3$COCH$_3$	56℃	20.7	任意	混溶
乙醇 C$_2$H$_5$OH	78℃	24.3	任意	混溶
甲醇 CH$_3$OH	64℃	33.6	任意	混溶
二甲基甲酰胺 HCON(CH$_3$)CH$_3$	153℃	37.6	任意	混溶
乙腈 CH$_3$CN	82℃	37.5	任意	混溶
乙二醇 CH$_2$CHCH$_2$OH	197℃	37.7	任意	混溶
甘油 CH$_2$OHCHOHCH$_2$OH	390℃	42.5	任意	混溶
甲酸 HCOOH	101℃	58.5	任意	混溶
水 H$_2$O	100℃	80.4	任意	混溶
甲酰胺 HCONH$_2$	211℃	101	任意	混溶
四氢呋喃	66℃	7.58	任意	混溶

注：有机溶剂多易燃，有害或有毒。

附表2　分离各类成分的溶剂系统和显色剂

化合物类型	溶剂系统	显色剂
脂肪酸及其酯类	乙醚 – 己烷 – 甲醇 （25：74：1）	50% H$_2$SO$_4$
	乙醚 – 己烷 （30：100）	
	二乙醚 – 石油醚 （5：95）	
	己烷 – 苯 （65：35）	
	己烷 – 苯 （5：5）	5% 邻钼酸的4%盐酸醇溶液
蜡质类	二乙醚 – 乙醚 （5：95）	
胆固醇类	石油醚 – 二乙醚 （4：1）	5% H$_2$SO$_4$
	二乙醚	
含氧脂肪酸	二乙醚 – 石油醚 （4：1）	
甾醇类	异丙醇 – 三氯甲烷 （1.5：98.5）	50% H$_2$SO$_4$
	三氯甲烷	
	己烷 – 乙醚 （4：1）	
	己烷 – 苯 （5：3）	
	石油醚 – 苯 （5：3）	
	石油醚 – 三氯甲烷 – 醋酸 （75：25：0.5）	
五环三萜	苯 – 5%盐酸	5% H$_2$SO$_4$和5%醋酐
	醋酸乙酯	
	苯	
单萜烃类	己烷	五氧化锑三氯甲烷溶液
	苯	

化合物类型	溶剂系统	显色剂
萜醇类	己烷 - 乙醚 (4:1)	
	己烷 - 苯 (5:3)	
	石油醚 - 三氯甲烷 - 醋酸 (75:25:0.5)	50% 硫酸三氯化锑三氯甲烷溶液
挥发油	己烷 - 乙酸 - 三氯甲烷 (6:2:2)	1% 香兰醛浓硫酸溶液
	甲苯 - 醋酸乙酯 (7:3)	
内酰胺衍生物	醋酸乙酯	碘
化合物类型	溶剂系统	显色剂
雌性激素	异辛烷 - 三氯甲烷 - 乙醇 (40:70:18)	50% 硫酸乙醇溶液
吡啶同系物		Dragendorff 试剂

附表 3　萃取水溶液用的溶剂[①]

	B. P. (℃)	可燃性[②]	毒性[③]	注
苯	80.1	3	3	易成乳浊液[③]；较适宜于从缓冲液中提取生物碱及酚类
2 - 丁醇	99.5	1	3	高沸点；较适宜于从缓冲液中提取高极性水溶性物质
四氯化碳	76.5	0	4	易干燥；较适宜于非极性物质
三氯甲烷	61.7	0	4	能形成乳浊液；易于干燥
二乙醚	34.5	4	2	能吸收大量水；优良的通用溶剂
二异丙醚	69	52	2	长期贮存后能形成爆炸性过氧化物；较适宜于从磷酸盐缓冲的溶液提取羧酸
乙酸乙酯	77.1	3	1	吸附大量水；很适宜于极性物质
Freon 11	24	0	1	各种 Freon 都很适宜于挥发性非极性化合物；较贵
Freon 113	47.7	0	1	
二氯甲烷	40	0	1	会形成乳浊液；易于干燥
正戊烷	36.1	4	1	烃类均易于干燥
正己烷	69	4	1	适用于极性物质
正庚烷	98.4	3	1	均为不良溶剂

①本表中的大部分数据取自 A. J. Gordon and R. A. Ford, The chemist's Companion (wileylnterscience, New York, 1972) 一书。

②4 代表最毒或最易燃。4 > 3 > 2 > 1；0 代表不燃。

③用有机溶剂萃取水溶液时会形成乳浊液，有可能使分离变得很困难，溶液呈碱性时，这种乳浊液更易形成；加稀硫酸 (如果许可) 可以破坏这种乳浊液。以下是通常使用的破乳法；将水相用盐饱和 ($NaCl$, Na_2SO_4 等)；加几滴醇或醚 (尤其当有机层是 $CHCl_3$ 时)；将混合物进行离心，这是最成功的方法之一。

附表 4　用于有机溶剂的中等强度的干燥剂

干燥剂	容量[①]	速率[②]	注
$CaSO_4$	$1/2H_2O$	极快 (1)	以商品名 Drierite 出售，加或不加颜色指示剂；非常有效，干时，指示剂 ($CoCl_2$) 呈蓝色，吸水后变成粉红色 (容量 $CoCl_2 \cdot 6H_2O$)；适用温度范围为 -50～86℃。某些有机溶剂能使 $CoCl_2$ 沥出或改变颜色 (如丙酮，醇类，吡啶等)
$CaCl_2$	$6H_2O$	极快 (2)	不很有效；只用于烃或卤代烃 (与含氮和含氧化合物形成溶剂化物，络合物，或发生反应)
$MgSO_4$	$7H_2O$	极快 (4)	较好的通用干燥剂；非常惰性但可能略呈酸性 (避免用于对酸极敏感的化合物)。可能溶于某些有机溶剂
4A 分子筛	高	快 (30)	非常有效；建议先用普通干燥剂后再用此物 (见下述有关分子筛的详情)。3A 分子筛也是较好的干燥剂

干燥剂	容量[①]	速率[②]	注
Na₂SO₄	10H₂O	慢（290）	非常温和，非常有效，便宜，高容量；很适于初步干燥，但不得使溶液受热
K₂CO₃	2H₂O	快	对于酯、腈、酮，特别对于醇，是良好干燥剂，不可用于酸性化合物
NaOH、KOH	极高	快	高效，但只适于用不会使它们溶解的惰性溶剂；特别用于胺
H₂SO₄	极高	极快	极为有效，但仅限于用来干燥饱和或芳香烃或卤代烃（硫酸会与烯或其他碱性化合物作用而使之损失）
氧化铝（Al₂O₃）或硅胶（SiO₂）	极高	极快	特别适宜于烃，应予研细；用过后将其加热（SiO₂为300°，Al₂O₃为500°）便可使之重新活化

①每摩尔干燥剂吸收水的摩尔数（最大量）。

②相对速率。前五行括号内的数字系指苯的相对干燥速率——数学小表示干燥快；溶剂改变时，吸水率低的干燥剂的次序会发生变化。[B. Pearson and Ollerenshaw, Chem., 370（1966）.]

附表5　用于有机液体的较强的去水剂

试剂[①]	与水形成的化合物	注
Na[②]	NaOH、H₂	用于烃和醚的去水很出色；但不能用于任何卤代烃。
CaH	Ca（OH）₂，H₂	最佳去水剂之一；比 LiAlH₄ 缓慢但效率相同且较安全。用于烃、醚、胺、酯、C₄ 和更高级的醇（勿用于 C₁，C₂，C₃ 醇），不得用于醛和活泼羰基化合物
LiAlH₄[③]	LiOH，Al（OH）₃，H₂	只适用于惰性溶剂［烃类、芳基卤（不能用于烷基卤），醚］；能与任何酸性氢和大多数官能团（卤、羰基、硝基等等）反应。使用时应小心；多余者可慢慢加入乙酸乙酯加以破坏
BaO 或 CaO	Ba（OH）₂或 Ca（OH）₂	慢而有效；主要适用于醇类和醚类，但不适宜于对强碱敏感的化合物
P₂O₃	HPO₃，H₃PO₄，H₄P₂O₇	非常快且高效，高度酸性。建议先经预干燥。仅适用于惰性化合物（尤其适用于烃、醚、卤代烃、酸、酐）

①最佳的去水剂应是能与水反应且不可逆的（且不与溶剂和溶质反应），它们也是极其危险的，故应先经不太剧烈的去水剂粗略干燥后才准许使用这类去水剂，这类去水剂几乎总是只在蒸馏溶剂之前或在蒸馏过程中对它进行去水。尽管 MgClO₄ 是最有效的干燥剂之一，但不予推荐，因为操作不慎会发生爆炸。

②J. T. Baker 公司出售一种称做 Dri-Na 的合金，含 Na 10%，Pb 90%；这种干的，粒状试剂只与空气慢慢反应，但其干燥醚等溶剂的效率与钠相同。

③另一种危险性较小，但效率相当的干燥剂是 Na（CH₃OCH₂CH₇O）₂AlH₂，称为 Vitride（Realco Chemical Campany 出品，可自 Eastman Kodak 公司购得）。

附录二　常用层析材料及有关数据表

层析法又称为色谱法，根据分离原理的不同可分为吸附层析、分配层析、葡聚糖凝胶层析和离子交换层析等。常用的层析材料有硅胶、氧化铝、活性炭、聚酰胺、硅藻土、葡聚糖凝胶、离子交换树脂等。以下是一些常用层析材料的数据。

附表6　一些固定相常用的调浆溶剂及其剂量

固定相	选用溶剂	固定相（g）：溶剂（ml）
硅胶 G	水	1：（1～2.5）
氧化铝 G	水	1：（1～3）
硅藻土 G	水	1：2
纤维素 G	水，95%乙醇或丙酮	1：（5～6）
聚酰胺	甲醇	1：（4～10）

附表 7　不同材料的薄层活化参考条件

固定相	活化温度/℃	活化时间/min
硅胶	110	60
纤维素	105	20～30
氧化铝	110	30
硅藻土	110	30
聚酰胺	60～80	30

附表 8　一些常用硅胶的孔结构参数

硅胶类型	比表面积/$m^2 \cdot g^{-1}$	比孔体积/$ml \cdot g^{-1}$	平均孔径/nm
1	675	0.68	4
2	462	0.46	4
3	550	0.82	6
4	500	0.75	6
5	315	0.73	9
6	420	1.05	10

附表 9　硅胶活度与含水量的关系

活度级	含水量（%）
I	0
II	5
III	15
IV	25
V	38

附表 10　氧化铝活度与含水量的关系

活度级	含水量（%）
I	0
II	3
III	6
IV	10
V	15

附表 11　葡聚糖凝胶吸水量与应用范围

型号	分离范围（分子量）		吸水量/$ml \cdot g^{-1}$	膨胀体积/$ml \cdot g^{-1}$	浸泡时间/h	
	蛋白质	多糖			室温	沸水浴
G-10	≥700	≥700	1.0±0.1	2～3	3	1
G-15	≥1500	≥1500	1.5±0.2	2.5～3.5	3	1
G-25	1000～5000	100～5000	2.5±0.2	4～6	3	1
G-50	1500～3万	500～1万	5.0±0.3	9～11	3	1
G-75	3000～7万	1000～5万	7.5±0.5	12～15	24	3
G-100	4000～15万	1000～10万	10±1.0	15～20	72	5
G-150	5000～40万	1000～15万	15±1.5	20～30	72	5
G-200	5000～80万	1000～20万	20±1.0	30～40	72	5

附表 12　常用离子交换纤维素的特征

名称	离子交换基	性质	交换容量（mmol/g）
CM - 纤维素	OCH_2COOH	弱酸性	0.62 ± 0.1
P - 纤维素	OPO_3H_7	中强酸性	$0.8 \sim 0.9$
Se - 纤维素	$OC_2H_4SO_3H$	强酸性	$0.2 \sim 0.3$
DETA - 纤维素	$OC_2H_4N（C_2H_5）_2$	强碱性	$0.4 \sim 0.55$
TEAE - 纤维素	$OC_2H_4N^+（C_2H_5）_3$	中强碱性	$0.55 \sim 0.75$
PAB - 纤维素	$OCH_2O_6H_4NH_2$	弱碱性	$0.15 \sim 0.2$
AE - 纤维素	$OC_2H_4NH_2$	弱碱性	0.33 ± 0.1
Ecteola - 纤维素	$CH_2CHOH - CH_2N^+（CH_2CH_2OH）_3$	弱碱性	$0.3 \sim 0.4$
BD - 纤维素	$OC_2H_4N（C_2H_5）_2$	中强碱性	0.8 ± 0.05
GE - 纤维素	$OC_2H_4NHC = NH_2NH_2{}^+Cl^-$	强碱性	$0.2 \sim 0.3$
BND - 纤维素	$OC_2H_4N（C_2H_5）_2$	中强碱性	0.8 ± 0.05

附表 13　常用葡聚糖凝胶离子交换剂的性能

类型	性质	交换容量	操作 pH 范围
DEAE - sephadex A - 25	弱碱性	$3 \sim 4$	$2 \sim 9$
DEAE - sephadex A - 50	弱碱减性	$3 \sim 4$	$2 \sim 9$
QAE - sephadex A - 25	弱碱性	$2.6 \sim 3.4$	$2 \sim 10$
QAE - sephadex A - 50	弱碱性	$2.6 \sim 3.4$	$2 \sim 10$
CM - sephadex A - 25	弱酸性	$4 \sim 5$	$6 \sim 10$
CM - sephadex A - 50	弱酸性	$4 \sim 5$	$6 \sim 10$
SP - sephadex A - 25	弱酸性	$2 \sim 2.6$	$2 \sim 10$
SP - sephadex A - 50	弱酸性	$2 \sim 2.6$	$2 \sim 10$

附表 14　几种国产滤纸的型号与性能

型号	标重（$g \cdot m^{-2}$）	厚度/mm	吸水性（30 min 内水上升高度/mm）	灰分/（$g \cdot m^{-2}$）	展开速度
1	90	0.17	$120 \sim 150$	0.08	快
2	90	0.16	$90 \sim 120$	0.08	中
3	90	0.15	$60 \sim 90$	0.08	慢
4	180	0.34	$120 \sim 150$	0.08	快
5	180	0.32	$90 \sim 120$	0.08	中
6	180	0.30	$60 \sim 90$	0.08	慢

附录三　NMR 谱测定常用氘代溶剂及其溶剂杂质峰和水峰的 ^1H 和 $^{13}C - NMR$ 图谱和数据

Name	b. p. （℃）	δ_H（mult）	δ_C（mult）
Acetone - d_6	57	2.04（5）	206.0（13） 29.8（7）

续表

Name	b. p. (℃)	δH (mult)	δC (mult)
Acetonitrile – d_3	82	1.93 (5)	118.2 (br.)
			13 (7)
Benzene – d_6	80	7.15 (br.)	128.0 (3)
Chloroform – d	62	7.24 (1)	77.0 (3)
Deuterium Oxide	101.4	4.63 (DSS)	
		4.67 (TSP)	
Diethyl – d_{10} Ether	35	3.34 (m)	65.3 (5)
		1.07 (m)	14.5 (7)
Dimethyl – d_6 Sulphoxide	189	2.49 (5)	39.5 (7)
Methyl Alcohol – d_4	66	4.78 (1)	49.0 (7)
		3.30 (5)	
Methylene Chloride – d_2	40	5.32 (3)	53.8 (5)
Pyridine – d_5	116	8.71 (br.)	149.9 (3)
		7.55 (br.)	135.5 (3)
		7.19 (br.)	123.5 (3)

^{1}H–NMR: H$_2$O PEAKS IN DEUTERATED SOLVENTS

^{1}H NMR Spectra of Common Solvents,
showing position of water peaks,
(δ in ppm relative to TMS)

CD$_2$Cl$_2$ Methylene Chloride–d_2 H$_2$O at 1.22 ppm
DCON(CD$_3$)$_2$ Dimetheyl formamide DMF–d_7 H$_2$O at 3.0 ppm
C$_5$D$_5$N   Pyridine–d_5 H$_2$O at 5.0 ppm
C$_6$D$_5$CD$_3$ Toluene–d_8 H$_2$O at 0.1–0.2 ppm

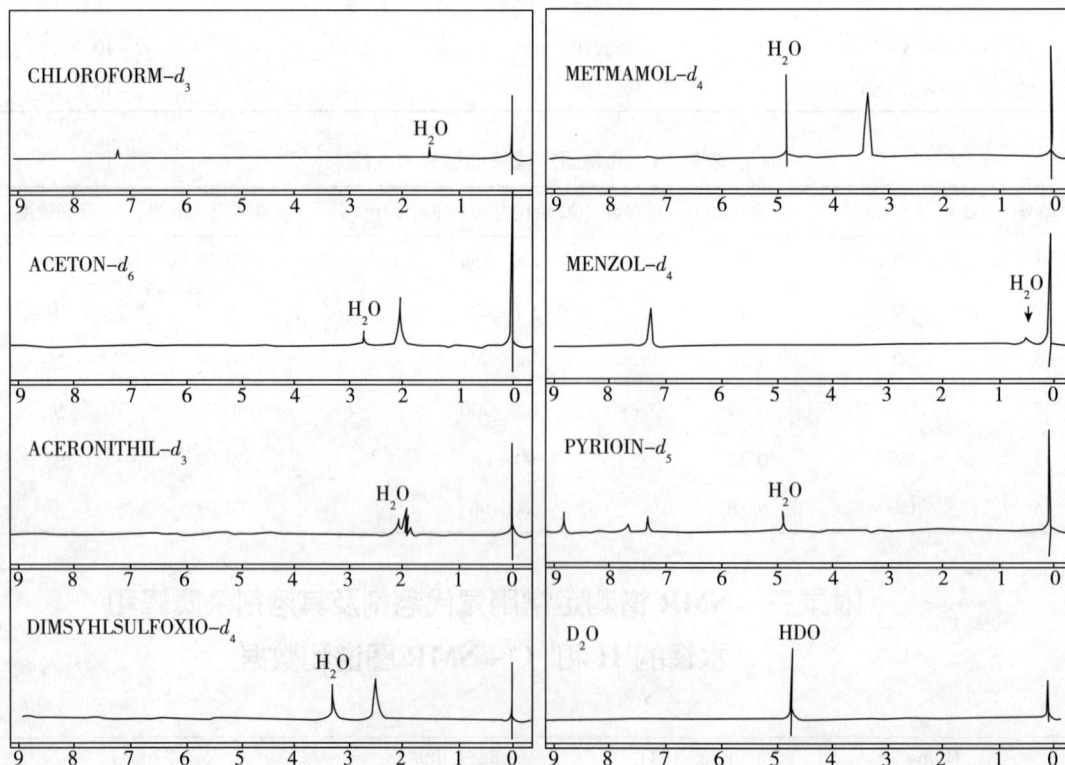

附录四　天然药物化学常用工具书、网络资源和期刊介绍

（一）常用工具书

1. 植物药有效成分手册　江纪武、肖庆祥编著，1986 年人民卫生出版社出版。

药用植物有效成分手册收载药用植物的天然活性成分 1375 个。各成分按英文名称字顺排序。其内容包括名称、异名、化学名、结构式、理化常数、光谱数据、植物来源、作用、用途及主要文献。资料较丰富，书后有六种索引，查阅非常方便。

2. The Merck Index（默克索引）　*An encyclopedia of chemicals drugs and biologicals*

最近版为 2000 年的第 12 版（每 8 年再版一次）。全书收载化学药物共 10014 条，按药品名称英文字母顺序排次。每一药品下有化学名、商品名、别名、分子式、分子量、元素百分比、参考文献（包括提取分离、结构、合成等）、结构式、化学和物理性质、衍生物、用途等内容。正文后有各种资料数据、药品、分子式及 CAS 登记号索引。

3. Dictionary of organic compounds（有机化合物辞典）　英国 Chapman and Hall 公司出版。J. Bucking-ham 主编，第五版（1982）。

《有机化合物辞典》习称《海氏有机化合物辞典》。自 1934—1936 年第一版以来，已有五十年的历史。这部著作为常见有机化合物结构、理化性质及重要文献的著名工具书。第五版 1982 年发行，约有 46000 个化合物条目，包括 15 万个化合物。主要内容共五本，按化合物名称的英文字母顺序排次。另有化合物名称索引一本，分子式、杂原子及 CAS 登记号索引一本。1983 年每年出版一本补充本，各补充本均附有各种索引，查阅非常方便。我国曾将 1953 年出版的第三版译成中文称《汉泽海氏有机化合物辞典》。

4. Hand book of Data organic Compound So vol. I. Ⅱ.　CRC 有机化合物数据手册，Robert C. Weast. Melvin J. Astle.

《CRC 有机化合物数据手册》新版 1985 年发行，其内容有 24415 个化合物，列表内容有本书编号、CAS 登记号、伯恩斯坦编号、名称、别号、分子式、分子量、nD、m. p.、bp.、d_4、$[\alpha]_D$、结晶性状、颜色、溶解度等。并有光谱文献、结构式以及各化合物溶点、沸点和分子式索引。

（二）有关天然药物化学研究的一般系统检索刊物

1.《中国药学文摘》　中药资料电脑检索中心、国家医药管理局科学技术情报研究所编辑。

1982 年，1983 年有试刊各一本，1983 年~1984 年 1-6 卷，每卷 6 期，每年有年度总索引（题目、作者及英文拉丁学名），国内发行。

2.《中文科技资料目录——中草药》　国家中医药管理局天津药物研究院，国家医药管理局中草药情报中心站编辑。

1978 年—1988 年 1-11 卷，每年各六期，并有年总索引（题目、作者）。

3. Abstracts of Chinese Medicines（ACME）　（an International Quarterly Abstracting Journal on Chinese Materia）张雄谋主编，香港中文大学中药研究中心出版。

《中药文摘》创刊于 1986 年 10 月，收集有关中医、中药、植物、化学的杂志刊物 140 余种的论文，本文摘内容有生药学、化学、药理学、毒理学、生物药剂学、临床报告、中西结合药物、综述等的文摘，以及专题综述文章。文摘后有拉丁文名称，拼音及一般英文

名称索引。

4. Chemical Abstracts（CA）（化学文摘） 美国化学文摘创刊于 1907 年，今（1988 年 7 月 12 日），已出版 109 卷。其内容见专著，专文介绍：美国《化学文摘》查阅法。澎海卿，化学工业出版社（1980）；化学通报，1980，（8）：508；（10）：632；药学通报，1981，16（2）：45（109）；16（12）：45（749）。

5. Index Chemicus（IC）（化合物索引） 化合物索引创刊于 1960 年，为周刊。至 1988 年开始为 111 卷第 10 期，1969 年前用"Index Chemicus"。1970 年改用"Current abstract of Chemistry and index Chemicus"。1987 年起改称"Index Chemicus"原名。

6. Chemical Titles（CT）（化学题录） 化学题录创刊于 1960 年，为双周刊，美国化学会出版。它收录理论化学、应用化学和化学工程及有关药学方面的资料，比美国化学文摘出版快 1~2 月。无累积索引，所报道的题录都会纳入随后出版的 CA 中。每期内容分为三部分即关键词前后关连索引，收载的期刊内容目录和作者索引。

7. Natural Product Reports（天然产物报告） 天然产物报告创刊于 1984 年，为双月刊，英国皇家化学会出版。它收录生物有机化学当代进展的综述论文，每期 2~10 篇不等，每卷后附有多种索引。

8. Natural Product Updates（最新天然产物） 创刊于 1988 年，为月刊，英国皇家化学会出版。它收录一些新的期刊杂志上刊载的新化合物文献结构式、名称、mp、$[\alpha]_D$、分子式、分子量，有的附有所用技术条件。并有新天然物来源、新书、新综述文以及会议记录等内容。附有作者、原植物来源资料、拉丁文来源、化合物分类及天然产物索引。这是为了解天然产物化学新研究进展的简要快报。

9. Biological Abstracts（BA）（生物学文摘） 美国生物学文摘创刊于 1926 年，由美国生物学文摘科学情报社编辑出版。该刊前身是细菌学文摘（1917~1925）和植物学文摘（1918~1926），1926 年合并后改用现名。从 1959 年起每半月出一期，1972 年每年二卷，每卷 12 期，每月 1、15 日出版。

生物学文摘是检索生物学、农学、医药学方面的文献资料的重要文摘之一，取材主要是期刊论文、论文集、技术报告、学位论文及图书等。

（三）常用搜索引擎

1. SciFinder Scholar SciFinder Scholar 是美国化学学会（ACS）旗下的化学文摘服务社 CAS（Chemical Abstract Service）所出版的《Chemical Abstract》化学文摘的在线版数据库学术版，前身是美国《化学文摘》。自推出以来，SciFinder 一直都是全世界的科学家进行化学课题研究、成果查阅、学术期刊浏览以及把握科技发展前沿的最得力工具。与 CA 相比，SciFinder 具有更丰富的内容和更强大的功能。SciFinder 数据库收录的文献资料来自全球 200 多个国家和地区，涉及 60 多种语言，包括 1 万多份期刊、63 家专利机构的专利、评论、会议录、论文、技术报告和图书中的各种化学研究成果。与其他科学资源相比，SciFinder 有更多的期刊和专利链接，能够帮助您在研究过程中更有效率，更有创意。

2. PubMed PubMed 系统是由美国国立生物技术信息中心（NCBI）开发的用于检索 MEDLINE、PreMED－LINE 数据库的网上检索系统。MEDLINE 是美国国立医学图书馆（U. S. National Library of Medicine）最重要的书目文摘数据库，内容涉及医学、护理学、牙科学、兽医学、卫生保健和基础医学。收录了全世界 70 多个国家和地区的 4000 余种生物医学期刊，现有书目文摘条目 1000 万余条，时间起自 1966 年。

3. Web of Science（SCI \ SSCI \ AHCI）　Web of Science 是全球领先的跨学科引文数据库，其中收录了 11,000 多种世界权威的、高影响力的学术期刊及全球 110,000 多个国际学术会议录，内容涵盖自然科学、工程技术、生物医学、社会科学、艺术与人文等领域，最早回溯至 1900 年。Web of Science 涵盖了全球最权威的三大引文索引数据库，包括自然科学引文索引 SCI，社会科学引文索引 SSCI 和人文艺术引文索引 AHCI。

Science Citation Index（科学引文索引，简称 SCI）是全球知名的科技文献检索工具，全球知名的引文索引数据库，因为其具有开创性的内容、高质量的数据以及悠久的历史使得 SCI 在全球学术界有极高的声誉。作为世界知名的引文索引数据库，SCI 包含的学科超过 170 个，收录了自然科学和工程领域内的 8000 多种高质量学术期刊近百年的数据内容，使用 SCI，能够轻松破解最新、最重要的科技文献在期刊与期刊之间、数据库与数据库之前以及出版社与出版社之间的壁垒，帮助科研人员能够轻松地找到世界范围内，自己研究领域最新、最相关、最前沿的科技文献，激发科研人员的研究思想，获取更多的研究思路。

Social Science Citation Index（社会科学引文索引，简称 SSCI）是全球著名的科技文献检索工具 Science Citation Index（科学引文索引，简称 SCI）的姊妹篇，是全球知名的专门针对人文社会科学领域的科技文献引文数据库。其内容覆盖了政治、经济、法律、教育、心理、地理、历史等五十多个的研究领域，收录 2400 多种学术期刊。在全球化一体化的今天，在东西方文化渴望进一步交流的今天，SSCI 是我们从事人文社会科学研究的重要工具。利用 SSCI 能够帮助广大社会科学的科研人员获得一个全新的视角去研究社会科学。

Arts & Humanities Citation Index（人文艺术索引，简称 A&HCI）与 SSCI 一样是 Web of Science 当中一个子库，是全球最权威的人文艺术引文数据库，内容涉及到人文艺术的各个领域，目前收录人文艺术领域 1,600 多种国际性、高影响力的学术期刊，数据最早可以回溯到 1975 年。其内容涵盖了哲学、文学、文学评论、语言学、音乐、艺术、舞蹈、建筑艺术、亚洲研究、历史及考古等学科。

（四）常用外文数据库

1. ACS 数据库　即 American Chemical Society（美国化学学会）美国化学学会成立于 1876 年，现已成为世界上最大的科技学会，会员数超过 163,000 人。多年以来，ACS 一直致力于为全球化学研究机构、企业及个人提供高品质的文献资讯及服务。秉持着服务大众、提升学者的专业素养、追求卓越的理念，ACS 在科学、教育、政策等领域提供了多方位的专业支持，成为享誉全球的科学出版机构。ACS 所出版的期刊有 37 种，内容涵盖了 24 个主要的化学研究领域。其期刊被 ISI 的 Journal Citation Report（JCR）评为"化学领域中被引用次数最多的化学期刊"。目前国内已经有近 80 个高校使用 ACS 网络版。

2. Elsevier 数据库　SDOS（Science Direct On Site）原名为 EES（Elsevier Electronic Subscriptions）。EES 自 1999 年 1 月起正式使用 SDOS 作为新名称，以确保 Elsevier Science Direct 一系列服务名称的一致性。SDOS 是全球最大的出版商，Elsevier 所提供的 1100 种电子期刊（包括 Pergamon、North – Holland 出版物）订阅服务。每年出版大量的学术图书和期刊，大部分期刊被 SCI、SSCI、EI 收录，是世界上公认的高品位学术期刊。

3. John Wiley 数据库　John Wiley & Sons Inc.（约翰威立父子出版公司）创立于 1807 年，是全球历史最悠久、最知名的学术出版商之一，享有世界第一大独立的学术图书出版商和第三大学术期刊出版商的美誉。Wiley InterScience 是 John Wiley & Sons Inc 的学术出版物的在线平台，提供包括：化学化工、生命科学、医学、高分子及材料学、工程学、数学及统计学、物理及天文学、地球及环境科学、计算机科学、工商管理、法律、教育学、心理学、社会学等 14 学科领域的学术出版物。该出版公司出版的学术期刊质量很高，尤其在化学化工、生命科学、高分子及材料学、工程学、医学等领域。目前出版的近 500 种期刊中，2005 年有一半以上被 SCI、SSCI、和 EI 收录。

4. Springer Link 数据库　JALIS 集团采购 Springer Link 电子期刊全文数据库。包括电子、医学、计算机等 11 个大类的 400 种期刊的电子全文，镜像点设在清华大学图书馆，电子全文为 PDF 格式，使用前必须安装 Acrobat Reader。

（五）常用国外杂志

1. Organic Letters（有机快报）　中文名《有机快报》，缩写 Org. Lett. 或 OL，是一本同行评审的科学期刊，1999 年由美国化学会第一次发行。该期刊的影响因子为 5. 862（2011 年）、6. 324（2013 年）。《有机快报》被以下的文献或机构的数据库收录：化学文摘社（CAS），大英图书馆，EBSCOhost，PubMed，SwetsWise，Web of Science。

2. Journal Of Natural Products（天然产物）　由美国化学会（American Chemical Society）和美国生药学会（American Society of Pharmacognosy）联合出版的一本药物化学及生药学类杂志。杂志于 1979 年创刊于美国芝加哥，每月出版一期。该杂志现已被 CAS，Scopus，EBSCOhost，British Library，PubMed，Ovid，Web of Science 及 SwetsWise 等多家数据库收录。

3. Journal of Medicinal Chemistry（药物化学杂志）　药物化学杂志发表的文章观点和书评为一月更新一次。2010 年起药物化学杂志发表在了 ACS 上。药物化学杂志的出版，有助于分子结构和生物活性或作用方式关系的理解研究。研究的一些特定区域是，包括设计，合成有生物活性的化合物；分子修饰；对结构进行生物学研究；数据分析结构的复合系列等。

4. Tetrahedron（四面体）　是一本登载有关有机化学的原创研究论文的期刊。该期刊的影响因子为 2. 817（2013 年）。该期刊上的很多篇文章都已经得到多次引用，根据 Web of Science 2008 年的统计，有七篇发表在该期刊上的文章引用次数超过 1000 次。

5. Tetrahedron Letters（四面体快报）　四面体快报最大化的发展了有机化学的传播，快报每周出版一次，包含了实验化学和理论化学中的结构，技术，发展，结论。快报出版的迅速，及时的使重要研究结果从世界各地迅速传递。通过互联网访问，快报提供当前的或是即将发表议题的内容列表和图形摘要，大大方便了用户的使用需求。

6. Phytochemistry Letters（植物化学快报）　植物化学快报可以快速报道所有天然产物方面的研究，包括天然产物的结构鉴定；中草药的分析评价，疗效，安全性及临床研究；天然产物的生物合成和化学改性；天然产物代谢化学及药理学；天然产物的遗传学等。

7. Fitoterapia（植物疗法）　植物疗法是收载药用植物和具有生物活性植物的杂志，杂志特色主要是七个方面：药用植物的有效成分鉴定；发展具有生物活性植物提取物的标准化方法；植物提取物的生物活性鉴定；植物提取物的靶向和活性机制识别；药用植物生物量的生产和基因组特征识别；具有生物活性天然产物的生物化学和化学信息；药用植物的历史，临床和法律地位。

8. **Planta Medica（药用植物）** 由德国（西德）药用植物研究会出版，内容主要涉及登载药用植物及植物成分方面的研究报告及简报，是天然药物化学传统经典期刊之一。

（六）常用国内杂志

1. **中国天然药物（Chinese Journal of Natural Medicines）** 《中国天然药物》是由中国药科大学、中国药学会共同主办的国家级药学学术期刊，2003 年 5 月创刊，双月刊，逢单月 20 日出版，国内外公开发行。几年来，在编委会与编辑部的共同努力下，CJNM 取得了中国精品科技期刊、中国科协精品期刊、RCCSE 中国权威学术期刊、中国高校优秀期刊、中国科学引文数据库 CSCD 核心期刊、北大中文核心期刊、中国科技论文统计源期刊荣誉。2008 年起 CJNM 与 Elsevier 集团合作，在 ScienceDirect 全文数据库平台上出版国际网络版，国际下载量占 67%，大大提高国际可见度与国际影响力；同时 CJNM 开始以国际化为目标，2010 年已逐渐改为英文版；同年期刊采用汤森路透 Scholarone 网上投审稿系统，审稿人及作者来自世界 20 多个国家和地区，加快了出版速度，提高了国际影响。2012 年，《中国天然药物》成为中国药学会主办期刊中首个进入 SCIE 的科技期刊。

2. **中国化学快报（Chinese Chemistry Letters）** 《中国化学快报》杂志（简称 CCL）创刊于 1990 年 7 月，是中国化学会主办，中国医学科学院药物研究所承办的核心刊物，由著名化学家梁晓天院士主编。内容覆盖我国化学研究全领域，及时报道我中国化学领域研究的最新进展及热点问题，本刊报道的是原始性研究成果，在《中国化学快报》发表通讯后，可以扩充内容在其它刊物上发表。本刊为 SCI 期刊，月刊，每期 112 页，16 开本，向国内外公开发行。

3. **天然产物研究与开发（Natural Product Research and Development）** 《天然产物研究与开发》为国家科委和新闻出版署批准的国内外正式公开发行的专业性学术月刊，是我国最早报道天然产物研究与开发的刊物。主要刊载具生物活性的天然产物以及药用动植物的研究与开发的创新性成果，尤其是天然产物的生物活性、作用机理、提取分离新方法，复杂混合物快速分离分析，天然产物的结构改造、生物合成及生物转化、合成新方法、构效关系研究、活性评价新手段，天然产物综合利用等，涵盖天然产物化学、生物化学、药学及分子生物学等领域。

4. **中国药科大学学报（Journal of China Pharmaceutical University）** 《中国药科大学学报》是由国家教育部主管、中国药科大学主办的药学类综合刊物，1956 年创刊，双月刊，96 页。国内外公开发行。中国药科大学学报以中国药科大学为依托，面向国内外，促进药学界的学术交流，为我国的药学事业现代化服务。中国药科大学学报主要刊登合成药物化学、天然药物化学、生药学、中药学、药剂学、药物分析、药物生物技术、药理学、药代动力学等学科的原始研究论著。

参考文献

［1］ Clark F. Most, Jr. Experimental Organic Chemistry ［M］. New York：John Wiley & Sons, 1988.

［2］ 郭伟强，张培敏，边平凤. 分析化学手册 ［M］. 北京：化学工业出版社，2016.

［3］ 于德泉，杨俊山. 分析化学手册：第七分册（核磁共振波谱分析）［M］. 北京：化学工业出版社，1999.

［4］ 杨云，张晶，陈玉婷. 天然药物化学成分提取分离手册（修订版）［M］. 北京：中国中医药出版社，2003.

［5］ 徐任生. 天然产物化学 ［M］. 北京：科学出版社，1997.

［6］ 国家中医药管理局《中华本草》编委会. 中华本草（第2卷）［M］. 上海：科学技术出版社，1999.

［7］ 吴立军. 天然药物化学 ［M］. 北京：人民卫生出版社（第四版），2006.

［8］ 国家中医药管理局《中华本草》编委会. 中华本草（第8卷）［M］. 上海：科学技术出版社，1999.

［9］ 中国科学院上海药物研究所植物化学研究室. 黄酮体化合物鉴定手册 ［M］. 北京：科学出版社，1981.